W9-BVI-554

EAT YOURSELF THIN:

Secrets of the

Harbor Island Spas

EAT
YOURSELF THIN
Secrets of the
Harbor Island Spas

BARBIE FILLIAN
AND
LIDA LIVINGSTON

Forward by Stuart Paskow
Executive Director, Harbor Island Spa

ILLUSTRATED

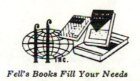

Fell's Books Fill Your Needs

FREDERICK FELL PUBLISHERS, INC.
NEW YORK, NEW YORK

Library of Congress Catalog Card No. 77-84426

ISBN 0-8119-0284-6

Copyright © 1977 by Barbie Fillian and Lida Livingston

All rights reserved. No part of this work covered by the copyright herein may be reproduced or used in any form or by any means—graphic, electronic, or mechanical, including photocopying, recording, taping, or information storage and retrieval systems—without the written permission of the publisher.

For information address:

Federick Fell Publishers, Inc.
386 Park Avenue South
New York, New York 10016

Published simultaneously in Canada by:
Thomas Nelson & Sons, Limited
Don Mills, Ontario, Canada

1 2 3 4 5 6 7 8 9 0

MANUFACTURED IN THE UNITED STATES OF AMERICA

TO STUART PASKOW
with heartfelt appreciation.
Barbie Fillian

●●●

TO LARRY and STUART PASKOW,
for proving, and helping others
prove, people can change and improve their lives.

Lida Livingston

Foreword

THE denial of food is never a permanent answer to the problem of obesity. When a person drastically restricts his/her food intake during a weight-loss campaign, the problem is: What happens when the dieter is let out of jail?

At Harbor Island Spa, our answer is—don't put the dieter into jail.

Diet control should not be a punishment. It should be—and we try to make it so—a pleasurable education. The Harbor Island Spa's original nutritional program was designed by the late, famous Norman H. Jolliffe, M.D., a physician internationally known for his work in the public health field, creator of New York's Obesity Clinic, and originator of the term "appestat" which explains the brain function that, when performing normally, automatically guides us into eating no more than our energy needs require. That's the real secret of weight control: the brain. Educate the brain to the need and desire to be trim, fit, and healthy, and the pounds will drop off and stay off.

We have added to and varied our diets and menus since they first were designed by Dr. Jolliffe. Barbie Fillian has made very important contributions, working with our chefs to create recipes that are as delicious as they are nutritious, and low in calories too. Barbie is dedicated to the happiness and well-being of our patrons and we were delighted when she responded to their oft-repeated requests for a book on the Harbor Island Spa program, including its menus and recipes.

The desire to be healthy is universal. All we ask is that you open your mind to your body and use our program to reward you with improved health and fitness.

Add years to your life, and life to your years—for the health of it.

Stuart I. Paskow,
Executive Director,
Harbor Island Spa
West End, New Jersey

Contents

EAT YOURSELF THIN:

Secrets of the

Harbor Island Spas

Chapter 1

Ten Commandments For A Healthy Appestat

YOU can lose weight. Easily. Painlessly. Pleasurably. The proof of that? The thousands, including many rich and many famous, who have found their healthier, happier, slimmer selves at the Harbor Island Spas by following the scientific methods detailed in this book to get fat off and keep it off.

Through the Harbor Island Spas' system, you will lose whatever weight you want to lose no matter how many times you have tried and failed before. And you won't be subjected to strenuous fasts, fad or crash diets, or diet pills. The Harbor Island Spas' method will make you happier, healthier, and more attractive than you have ever been, and you will accomplish it all while eating delicious meals, including tasty desserts, snacks, and, if you wish, an occasional cocktail.

Starting on page 126, you'll find recipes from Harbor Island Spas—and complete nutritionally sound menus that will benefit you and every member of your family regardless of each individual's present or desired weight.

Thousands, including celebrities, jet setters, business executives, scientists, and homemakers too, have spent many thousands of dollars to lose weight at the Harbor Island Spas. You can achieve the same happy results for the mere price of this book—plus application of the principles and techniques, of course. How much can you lose? As much as you want for optimum fitness, and you can keep it off with ease. Admittedly not all do, but that's solely because they really haven't that great a desire to maintain their "ideal" weight.

The late comedian Jackie Leonard, for instance, visited Harbor Island Spa for four to six weeks annually and regularly lost 35 pounds, a weight loss he would maintain as long as he was in New York. Then, hitting the road, the weight rapidly went back on again.

"I've lost more weight than you weigh," he would mourn to the Spa's owner, and then would add in explanation: "I'm fine until I hit Chicago. Chicago does me in. I eat, drink, and gain weight."

Comedian Marty Allen dropped 40 pounds at Harbor Island Spa, going from 230 to his stabilized 190. He maintains his weight wherever he is simply by following our easy diet.

Meg Griffin, film star Debra Paget's delightful, ebullient sister, lost more than 100 pounds, and has kept it off. Debra, a Harbor Island Spa visitor with her sister, was never interested in losing weight but enjoyed the Harbor Island Spa's "plain, delicious" meals, massages, and exercise program.

The summer of 1976 brought a former famous Olympic star to us, with her dynamic husband. She is as chic today as when she was setting world swimming records and winning countless hearts. She and her husband are examples of what good diet, lots of tennis, swimming, and dancing can do to maintain vibrant health. Their long stay was, in part, to lose a few unwanted pounds. She dropped the six pounds in the first 10 days—all she wanted to lose—while her husband lost 16 in the same period.

"Everyone benefits from periodic pampering and absence of decision making," she said, "and that's what I find fun. Besides, it gives me great satisfaction to know I can go to parties and stay on a regimen of 600 calories a day."

Brilliant performers Steve Lawrence and Eydie Gorme, who early in their career entertained at the Spa, said, when they were at our Miami Spa while appearing at the Diplomat, that they enjoyed the "privacy and the discipline," the diet, massages, and exercise, and awareness that they were in top shape for their demanding two shows nightly. A performer cannot afford to be, or feel, ill.

Actress-singer Petula Clark has been a frequent Spa visitor, restricting her diet to 1000 calories a day to reduce only a few pounds in weight, and that slowly. Syndicated columnist Earl Wilson, whose famous chroniclings of the activities and comments of the world's celebrities require that he and his B.W. (Beautiful Wife) Rosemary dine out virtually nightly, calls the Spa his "escape hatch," where he's free from all pressures, including the temptation of rich food.

16

A well-known composer-singer-personality said the "music comes clearer" when he has lots of hours for tennis, and the food is "simple and I don't have to think about it." Weight is something he never has to think about.

The late opera star Richard Tucker vacationed regularly at Harbor Island Spa, not to lose weight, since he maintained an 1800-calories-a-day diet, but to go on a program of daily massage, relaxation, and exercise to keep his body and golden voice in peak condition for his challenging Metropolitan Opera roles. Throughout his life his voice retained its magnificence of tone and timbre.

"Harbor Island Spa," he would say, "is the only place I can go for a vacation that I don't go home needing a vacation."

Comedian Buddy Hackett has lost "hundreds of pounds" at Harbor Island Spa but concedes his focus is "too much on people and parties" to keep it off "until I start traveling with my own chef."

Comedienne Totie Fields maintains she lost weight at Harbor Island Spa, but between visits she always has returned to her old habits, induced not a little by the fact that her weight has been a staple of her comedic career. Now, with the tragedy of having lost a leg to diabetic complications behind her, the *new* Totie Fields has weight control as a prime goal in life and she has health as an all-important bonus. Effervescent Totie spends no time in self-pity; she's too busy enjoying the challenge of developing her new career.

Broadway-film actress-mimic Mae Questel, TV's Aunt Bluebelle, who was the model and voice for Betty Boop, the voice of Olive Oyl, and other famous cartoon characters, including, on occasion, Popeye himself, is a frequent visitor to Harbor Island Spa "for a rest," as well as to keep her weight stabilized at "pleasingly round." It is a fallacy to believe that everyone should be "standard thin." Besides the difference made by bone structure, there are many other individual differences that can put one person's "ideal" weight at 130 pounds, whereas another person of the same height and appparent bone structure feels better at 115.

Whether you want to lose 100, 50, 10, as few as five pounds, or no pounds at all or even gain a few, the Harbor Island Spa system of relaxation, exercise, and good simple food will work for you.

There are three basics in the Harbor Island Spa system of weight

17

loss/weight control: your desire, your diet, and exercise, and the most important of these is your desire, because from that all else stems. How much weight you lose and how fast you lose it depends very much on you—what you weigh now, your willingness to change certain habits that have put the weight on, and other factors unique to you, particularly why you have decided to lose.

You must forgo negativism. You must stop being despondent about being fat. Stop believing you will always be fat. Stop attributing your fat to your glands, to your mother, your father, your heredity in general; or, if you're a mother, to your last baby.

Believe it. Your fat comes from your head. Not from your stomach. Once you can accept that, you have taken another giant step toward achieving your ideal weight. The question you probably are asking is: How can I give up eating food when I enjoy food so much? You won't give up food. You will simply substitute other delicious food for the food you are now eating. You must eat, and well; perhaps better than you ever have before.

And you must *see* yourself slim. You must picture yourself not as obese—not as a person who has problems bending over to pick up something off the floor. Even if you are now *that* fat, you must picture yourself as ideal in shape; picture yourself as attractive, vital, vibrant. You must work on improving your self-image. To that end, you must picture yourself as worthy, as important, as successful, as loved. Those mental pictures will help you lose weight.

I wish each of you could join us at a Harbor Island Spa—in Miami or in New Jersey—but, since that's not possible, it is a pleasure to be able to share with you our famous and effective Harbor Island Spa secrets.

The key to losing weight is to restore your appestat to health. What's the appestat?

The appestat are cells in the midbrain that control how much you eat. Hunger is, indeed, in your head! "Appestat" was coined by the late Norman Jolliffe, M.D., founder of New York's famed Obesity Clinic and creator of Harbor Island Spa's nutritional program. The word dramatizes the relationship between caloric intake and energy output. It's a composite of appetite and "stat" (control). When normal and healthy, the appestat automatically balances the intake of food calories against their expenditure so that your weight remains stable, year after year.

How do you create a healthy, normal appestat?

By eating. By providing the cells and tissues of the midbrain with a good environment, and that's done by food—and exercise. A healthy environment requires that you eat a fully balanced diet, fats and carbohydrates as well as protein, vitamins, and minerals; that you drink plenty of water, and that you exercise.

You may walk, go dancing, play tennis, golf, swim, skin dive, ski, jog. Whatever pleases you. Setting-up exercises or Yoga aren't required. They are simply an efficient way to make sure you are exercising all the muscles you want to exercise in minimum time—including those of the face. So, for the sake of your looks as well as your appestat, remember that muscles that aren't exercised become flabby—atrophy. That includes the inner muscles and tissues too, which means your diet must include a certain amount of bulk and fiber foods to allow activity for those inner muscles and tissues as they process what you eat. While weight loss is not the prime reason for exercise, lack of exercise can make you fat. Look to the animal world for proof of that. When farmers want to fatten cattle, hogs, and geese for butchering, they feed extra rations of course, but they also confine the animals so they can't exercise. And exercise does burn up some calories. For example:

One hour of walking uses up 210 calories; one hour of golf, 250 calories; one hour of swimming, 300 calories; one hour of tennis, 420 calories.

Richard Tucker's habit of daily massage is something we all would benefit from. While it's not something we can do for ourselves, we all can learn massage techniques. Where husband and wife give each other massages—well, that can bring a new degree of pleasure and mutual appreciation into any marriage.

"Laying on of hands" is a reality in healing. The energy flow from one individual to another can make anyone feel better. Perhaps none of us was sufficiently stroked as a baby! We appreciate the touch as well as the energy flow—and the superb sense of serenity and relaxation imparted by massage.

Many of the celebrities who come to the Spa do not have a weight problem but they are concerned—as we all should be—about keeping in top health and appreciate that rest, relaxation, exercise, and superior nutrition are basic to that. Englebert Humperdinck, for instance, who stayed at the Spa during his engagement at Garden State Center in New Jersey's Holmdel , wanted what he got: privacy; good, simple nutritious food; the sea, the pool, and lots of opportunities for exercise; and massage to take the kinks out before or after performances.

When Barbra Streisand came to the Spa, she, then a brand new mother and admittedly addicted to ''junk food,'' wanted a complete change, including a planned diet and exercises to put her body swiftly back into optimum condition.

Doctors often say an ''active woman'' need not exercise after a baby's birth. Untrue! But a new mother should be aware of how to exercise to restore her organs to normal position most rapidly. You will find four simple procedures in the chapter on Exercising—as well as general exercises for men, women, and teen-agers. Everyone should exercise throughout life. If a serious problem exists, check with your doctor first.

As a nutritionist, I must interject that nursing helps restore the uterus to position and medical research shows that babies that are nursed are less likely to become obese and less likely to develop juvenile diabetes, too often a companion to obesity. Even a nursing mother can restrict her diet to 1200 nutritionally beneficial calories daily. If she is nursing her baby, she should, though, drink at least a quart of milk, plus juices, daily. My other recommendations include a low-sodium diet (because fluids tend to accumulate during pregnancy); small, frequent meals; limited intake of citrus fruits and juices and tomato juice, fruit juices diluted half-and-half with water; unlimited intake of carrot and green vegetable juices: restricted or no intake of coffee and tea; and a planned program of exercise and ''getting out'' to keep up the energy and spirits.

Developing a ''merry heart'' is a good goal for all of us and you can create much of our happy Spa atmosphere right in your own home. For instance, we always have music at our dinner meals—happy, pleasant dance music. No rock! If you have a record player, it's easy to select a program of records to play during your dinner meals. You'll reap several benefits:

Your family and/or guests will feel happier. You'll find you eat more slowly and therefore, normally, less. You may even dance. If your dining room is carpeted but you have a play, game, or

20

recreation room with wood or other hard surface, consider setting up a dining table there for at least one dinner a week. Dancing will perform miracles for your spirits, your digestion, and your suppleness. Look at Ray Bolger, the great dancer-comedian who created those immortal characters of the Scarecrow in M-G-M's *The Wizard of Oz* and *Charley's Aunt.* Now in his seventies, Ray Bolger makes it a habit to dance two hours every day. Result: his body movements are as free and limber as a 20-year-old's.

One of our permanent Spa guests is a great lady, Mrs. Louis Waronoff, former owner of a successful New York City dress shop, who, though now nearly 80, on the dance floor gives no impression of age at all.

"Dancing and diet keep me young," she smiles. "When I came here two years ago, I weighed too much. I felt breathless and, well, stuffed. Then, while eating better than I ever had eaten before, I lost 10 pounds and feel just wonderful."

She looks wonderful too, and recently has taken to entertaining at the Spa, singing, and often sings at New Jersey events. She's wearing beautiful gowns she designs and makes herself.

"I always wanted to sing but never took the time for lessons until I retired," she said. "I'm sure the teacher, when she first met me, thought she'd just indulge me, letting me try out for her. After she heard me sing, she said 'I'm surprised. I'll be pleased to have you as a pupil.' "

Mrs. Woronoff is learning to play the piano too, and participates in exercise classes daily.

"Keep busy. Keep trying new things. That's the secret," she said.

The greatest weight loss for a single week chalked up at Harbor Island Spa was by an important business executive who dropped 29½ pounds within 10 days of checking in to our New Jersey Spa. But he started at a weight of 319! For the past two years, he has been enjoying a healthy, stabilized weight of 200 pounds. He looks and feels great.

It is feasible, literally, to eat yourself thin—and, of course, to improve your health immeasurably in the process.

Mr. and Mrs. Max Kaufman, parents of famed New York disc jockey Murray the K, came to our New Jersey Spa to live in 1973 when Mr. Kaufman retired from his leather company. Both were overweight although neither was fat. But today they "feel wonderful."

"We really appreciate what the medically sound diet has done for us," Mr. Kaufman comments.

He has lost 20 pounds; she, 15, and they feel their present weights are what they'll remain at the rest of their lives.

Another business man moved to the Spa in 1974 after the death of his wife. Founder of a nationally known mortgage company, he was nearly 90. Weight was not his problem, but he was "run down and waiting to die." Today he has "rejuvenated arteries," has found a new dancing partner, and is enjoying life. "The right diet and good exercise make it fun to be alive," he said, and added with a twinkle, "and a good dance partner certainly helps."

Everyone at the Spa, beginning with Larry Paskow, the founder, is a firm believer that "age is in the mind," and we have many long-time guests who are firmly imbued with the same theory. Such a one is a beautiful lady in her late eighties. Widowed five times, she is still a charmer with an assortment of suitors. Whenever you see her, she is delightfully dressed in lovely nontraditional pastels—subtle violets, tawny pinks, imaginative blues that flatter her fair skin and her pretty, beautifully coifed blonde hair.

"Activity, that's the answer," she smiles, "and simple diet. When I come to the Spa, for the first three days I eat the same thing at breakfast, lunch, and dinner—generally only chicken. The pounds—five at least—fall away, and I'm ready for Barbie's mixed, low-calorie maintenance diet."

This Spa visitor has been wearing a size 10 ever since she was 18.

"I don't believe in thinking about the years," she comments, "but I do believe one should make an effort not to be a blight on the landscape."

Far from a blight, she's a decided visual asset, whether seen at breakfast wearing an indigo-blue silk pants suit or at dinner in a long, amber chiffon gown, necklaces, and earrings.

"Dressing for dinner is good for everyone's morale," she says crisply. "Dressing like a slob can lead to thinking like a slob and that leads to mental and physical decay."

Here are more of our "case histories":

When Meg Griffin first came to Harbor Island Spa in 1968, she weighed 235 pounds. Her dress size was 26½. She stayed, that first time, three months and lost 47 pounds. She has kept up her regimen of good diet and exercise over the years. Today she weighs 140 pounds; wears a size 14 dress and she is happier, healthier, and busier than she's ever been, contributing many hours of volunteer service to a Houston hospital each week.

Mona B. of Providence, R. I., checked into Harbor Island Spa weighing 299 pounds and wearing a size 27 dress. She lost 50 pounds during a four-week stay. She is continuing to lose steadily on a diet that ranges from 1000 to 1200 calories a day. Her goal is to weigh 130 for her five feet six inches.

Rosalind and Roy L., a New York couple in their forties, came to Harbor Island Spa in May 1974 for a long weekend. Both were overweight. He weighed 200 pounds at five foot seven. Rosalind, five foot two, was, when she came to us, so fat she refused to get on the scales. She said, "Just put it down that I can't get into a size 14 dress."

This couple has been with us frequently since that first weekend when they started the program that has allowed them to achieve their "ideal" weights. Rosalind, who is big-boned, has stabilized her weight at 122, but she now wears size 8 in slacks and size 10 in dresses and coats. Her husband has gone down to 155 pounds and has dropped so much from his waist that now he and she can exchange blue jeans!

Instead of bread they eat artichoke bread sticks. They rarely eat red meat today. They have learned to enjoy vegetables, raw and cooked. They have eliminated cold drinks with their meals.

Mrs. Claire D., married and the mother of three, had a lifelong tendency to nibble incessantly whenever she was depressed. When she learned her son was gravely ill, her nibbling became nearly nonstop. Her weight rose steadily but she continued to be a "chain eater" even though she knew her changed appearance was upsetting her entire family, and most particularly her ill son who blamed himself for her obesity.

During a crucial point of his illness, and his absence from home, Mrs. D. checked into the Spa with her teen-age daughter. Mrs. D. tells her story willingly:

"It was the festive atmosphere that helped me first," she said. "The dance music at dinner was delightful—just wonderful therapy.

It took me out of myself and made dieting less depressing.

"My daughter and I participated in the exercise classes, swam in the indoor pool, and for me each day was topped off with a body massage. For the first time in months I found I was sleeping without having to take a sedative. That first night at dinner, when Barbie sat with us and discussed the weight loss I wanted to achieve, she suddenly touched my daughter's hand.

"'Do you want to be fat?' Barbie asked.

"Looking at me with ill-concealed distaste, she exploded, 'Certainly not!'

"'Then you best learn to eat more slowly,' Barbie said. 'Fast eating is a very bad habit all fat people share in common. Fast eating can be the very first step on the path to fat.'

"My daughter laid down her fork. 'That's right,' Barbie said. 'Lay down your fork after every mouthful. That will force you to eat more slowly.'

"During our first visit to the Spa I attended every lecture on nutrition that was given, and I acquired a new haircut and makeup in the Spa's beauty shop. As soon as I felt lighter in weight, I felt lighter of heart. Today I wear size 10—not the size 14 pants I did when I first checked into the Spa, and shopping for clothes is fun again. With the exercise, the good food, and a happier attitude, my skin became well, glowing, and my hair started to shine as it has not since I was a teen-ager.

"I returned home just a day ahead of my son. His smile and look of pride told me it was all well worth the effort. I know my improved appearance and my happier, more relaxed manner have been a tremendous help to him. He made up the year he lost from school through illness, and recently was graduated from the university *magna cum laude*. Today my son has regained health completely once again."

Many who check into the Spa desire to gain weight. But some of the thin are fighting fat too.

One evening I was called to the table of a Maryland dentist and his very thin, very chic, very tense wife. The dentist asked me to suggest a weight-loss diet for his wife. Hiding my surprise, I sat down with them and during the next half-hour learned the wife was in a panic about weight. She took diet pills and she lived on a starvation diet, one she already was paying for in the form of tension and a

24

haggard face. I banished the dentist and went with his wife to their room. Then we talked and I knew victory was certain when, nearly three hours later, she opened her bottle of diet pills and flushed them down the toilet.

Her story: her best friend was a size 6. She wanted to be a size 6 too. Once she could be convinced that her goal should be to express her own individuality, she became willing to listen to what it meant to eat well and enjoy it. Over the next four months, she developed into a perfect size 10. The tension went from her face. Her complexion became radiant. She emanated happiness. So did the dentist.

"Our marriage has never been as happy as now," he said, on a return visit a few months later. "That includes in the bedroom too."

His wife laughed and said demurely, "We're happy." Then she opened her eyes wide and let out a burst of laughter. "More than happy. We just never dreamed we could have it so good."

Friends and scales are the dieters' worst enemies. Friends commiserate with you in the early days when you are struggling to feel content on a 1000- or 800-calories-a-day diet. They try to coax you to have a forbidden sweet, or even suggest you abandon the entire project. Friendship? One wonders.

No one should weigh him/herself every day. Once a week is plenty.

So many factors can affect the scales adversely and induce disappointment. If you've been carefully holding down your caloric intake and step on the scales one morning to discover your weight has gone up, you're apt to think, "What's the use?" and go out and have a chocolate sundae to comfort yourself.

The water content of the body is the chief factor in the erratic behavior of the scales. Human water content can vary from 45.6 per cent up to 75 percent. On the average, men's bodies contain about 10 percent more water than women's. But the water content of the body is not constant. A man weighing 150 pounds may contain as much as 81 pounds of solids: proteins, fats, carbohydrates, minerals. Or he may contain only 45 pounds of solids. If he weighs 150 pounds one day and 155 pounds the next, the solid material is likely to be exactly the same but the water content has swung from 93 to 98 pounds.

People who tend toward fat tend also toward unstable water content, their thirst mechanism having gone awry along with their appestat. When there is a dramatic weight loss over a few days, elimination of water is usually the reason. That was the case of our seven-day-weight-loss champion, a vice-president of Ford Motor Company. When he checked into the Spa weighing 319 pounds, his medical doctor in Detroit telephoned and told me to put him on a diet of 400 calories a day. I refused. When a great deal of weight is to be lost, it simply isn't wise to cut down caloric intake too abruptly or drastically. The doctor then suggested 600 calories. Refusing again, I said, "No less than 1000 calories to start."

Eventually I did reduce his caloric intake to 800 calories a day. Three months later, when he was preparing to leave the Spa 75 pounds lighter, I gradually shifted him up to 1200 calories a day. He had lost 12 inches from his waist, along with the weight.

Over the December holidays he gained six pounds—too many parties. He returned to us for a long weekend in January and shed 10 pounds. He stays on our diet now. His stabilized weight of 200 pounds is excellent for his height. build, and activity pattern.

Because the water content of the male is normally higher than that of a female, men tend to lose weight more rapidly than women. The male's No. 1 motivation for going on a diet is fear of a heart attack or, having survived one, determination to prevent another. When men do reduce, they find such side benefits as renewed energy, renewed interest in the opposite sex, renewed interest in everything in life—a broader range of vision instead of one that, previously, usually had focused on a single thing—generally business. And that business, they have found, generally becomes better when they become thinner, happier, and more relaxed—less compulsive.

One of our successes had a massive heart attack the night he arrived at the Spa. His wife was with him, and within minutes he was in the hospital under intensive care. As soon as food was allowed, his wife arranged that I supervise his diet. I designed one that would both reduce his weight and build up his system. When the acute stage was over, he was brought in an ambulance to the Spa. He and his wife remained with us all summer and continue to return to us each summer. They both feel and look fit. They come back to the Spa because they enjoy it. They stay on our diet at home too, knowing that a well-balanced diet is the way to stay healthy—that a good diet truly does add years to life and life to years.

A New York woman in her sixties came to the Spa on doctor's orders. Her triglycerides were exceedingly high. She was deeply frightened; ''sure'', she'd ''had it.'' During the six weeks she was at the Spa, she became entirely normal in all areas, including the triglycerides, and she'd lost 30 pounds.

But my first job was to help her overcome her panic so that she could believe she could recapture her health. I did that by recountng case history after case history of persons who arrived at the Spa thinking they were at death's door and who found that not only weren't they dying but now were feeling healthier and happier than in memory.

Anyone who is fat is bitter about it.

The fat ''jolly'' person is a myth. They may be laughing on the outside but they're crying on the inside.

Every fat person I've met—and I know thousands—is self-conscious about it. In lecture halls and exercise classes they take places in the back of the room. I try to keep those at the Spa from doing that. In every way possible, I try to make them appreciate they are important, valuable people. Once they can assume a sense of value—and it is assumed in the beginning—they're on their way to a thinner self. In time—and few notice when the change takes place— the assumption becomes the reality and that's cause for celebration, for I know then that their goal of losing weight and keeping it off will be achieved.

The tendency to fat often begins in the womb. There are still women who believe ''eating for two'' requires an upswing in caloric intake and they often add those calories with fats and carbohy-drates—''empty'' calories. The woman who wants a bright healthy baby should pay strict attention to the quality of what she eats, eliminating all the ''garbage,'' reducing her sugar and salt intake, and making sure that her meals are balanced and most particularly that she is taking in sufficient protein. Medical researchers state unequivocally that a deficiency of complete protein in the diet of a pregnant woman can limit the growth of the baby's brain. A baby's brain achieves some 80 percent of its growth during its first three years of life—including the nine months in the womb.

Children pay for their parents' mistakes and the food department is likely to be where they pay the highest. Parents should make sure their children have a varied, nutritionally sound diet, but

27

they also should stop teaching children to "clean your plate." They should not nag them to eat and they should not nag them not to eat if they are fat. It only worsens the situation. Nagged sufficiently, a child feels unloved, unworthy, and eats all the more—compulsively.

A boy, 11, who spent a summer with us, is a case in point.

Since babyhood, he'd been fat. His mother told me she had been very proud of her "fat, handsome baby." She, as many parents do, equated fat babies with healthy babies. Thin babies, ordinarily, are the healthy ones, suffering fewer colds, less mucous, fewer respiratory problems, less colic, fewer stomach upsets. Frequently they are completely free of all these things, simply growing up healthy. Fed well from birth and with no fuss ever made over food, they exemplify how a healthy appestat is created and maintained.

Our fat 11-year-old was depressed, lethargic, and preferred to stay buried in a book rather than join in sports or games. As we talked out his problems, he said over and over:

"My mother nags me about how much I eat."

At the Spa, with meals put in front of him without comment, he suddenly was finding that he liked to talk at meal time—instead of just gulping food—and he was surprised to find he wasn't hungry even though the portions were small. And suddenly he began participating in sports and exercise and swim classes. His smiles became sunny and spontaneous. He was a changed child—and so proud when, one day, he had to buy new jeans. His pants were falling off.

It was a bit tricky explaining to his mother that her worthy intentions were very bad therapy. I said, as gently as I could:

"Ignore what he eats. Ignore his diet. Don't speak about it. Just let him know how much you appreciate him; how much you love him. Let him know you have confidence he can solve any problem he'll ever have, including his present one of excess weight. Then, please, don't mention weight to him ever again."

She looked at me silently, steadily, for what seemed minutes. Then she said. "All right. I'll leave him in your hands."

A question I'm regularly asked is, "When you've never been fat, how can you know how I feel?"

And I reply honestly, "Because I know thousands of you and inevitably have found the same feelings—the same deep-seated unhappiness with self, or that an upsurge in problems has driven you to eat as solace.''

Enjoyment of food is a basic cause of fat, of course. But more often tension and frustration are the cause. Some people, when they are tense and nervous, lose their appetite completely but, from my experience, more eat compulsively, not even noticing that they are doing so.

Alice K., now 60, a widowed grandmother residing in New England, came from a family of hearty eaters. Alice's mother and grandmother were celebrated as bakers and believed in setting a ''bountiful table.'' Alice was a fat child, a fatter teen-ager, but finally, rebelling at teasing from classmates, started on her first diet at 14, totally ignoring her mother's complaints she wasn't ''eating enough to keep a bird alive.''

Over the years Alice tried just about every kind of diet invented—single-food diets, high-protein diets, the Weight Watchers diet, which she concedes could have worked except that she ''couldn't be bothered with weighing everything.''

In 1963, en route to Colombia for a month-long holiday, she developed a severe pain in her face that she thought was a toothache. The pain was so severe she left the airplane in Miami and consulted a dentist. He could find nothing wrong with her teeth. But the pain continued, so she returned to her home in Boston. But let her tell it:

''Nineteen doctors later, including psychiatrists, I checked myself into a hospital in Boston and demanded that I be given every test possible. My pain, I maintained, was not a creation of my imagination. Besides, I was losing the hearing in one ear.

''It was over a week before the cause was located: a tumor on a nerve. During the year from the beginning of the pain until the diagnosis and removal of the tumor in the hospital, I had been eating compulsively—from sheer frustration. I had gone from my normal weight of 145 pounds to 198.

''After my recovery from the operation I tried to diet, but instead of losing I gained. When I tipped the scales at 210, my doctor suggested that I needed a 'protected environment' and continuing guidance until I reversed the trend and brought my weight down significantly. I checked into Harbor Island Spa—and stayed three months. Barbie Fillian helped me with my diet, and I joined the Spa's exercise classes. It was difficult in the beginning—not the

29

reduction of food to 800 calories a day, but development of faith that I really could get down to a decent weight. I was like an inflated balloon—all of a width from bust to thighs, no waistline at all.

"Then I began to glimpse an indentation above my hips and then I could see that my legs were much slimmer, from hips to feet. It was exciting! I joined more exercise classes—even a dance exercise class!.

"I never felt hungry. Instead, I found that I was enjoying each meal immensely—far more than before, because I was enjoying the flavors and combinations and eating desserts with a clear conscience. My happiest day in years was when I decided my dresses were just too sloppy; and when I went into the store, I discovered I was down to size 14."

Before she left for her home, Alice had lost 39 pounds. She kept on with our diet at home and over the next three months she continued to lose, but the rate was slowed because she had increased her caloric intake to 1000 a day. Eventually, however, she returned to the 145 pounds that, for her, is "ideal." She went to parties and found no problem in refraining from overindulgence in food, and she continued with her exercise program. Although she never regained the hearing in her damaged ear, she feels "well content," and delighted that she requires no medications at all.

When fat people ask for proof that the Harbor Island Spa program will not only get fat off but keep it off, I point to Larry Paskow, founder of Harbor Island Spa in Miami in 1951, and his son, Stuart, president of the New Jersey Harbor Island Spa, founded in 1956.

Larry Paskow was a major investor in Vitamin Corporation of America that Dr. Jolliffe, a pioneer in megavitamin therapy, headed as president. The two were close friends and Dr. Jolliffe regularly chided Larry Paskow about his weight—280 pounds, although spread over a six-foot-four-inch frame.

Finally Dr. Jolliffe managed to get Larry Paskow onto a program of diet and exercise designed to put his appestat back into order. In the six months it took to drop 80 pounds from his body and six inches from his waist, Larry Paskow developed a new resolve: to sell his interests in Vitamin Corporation of America and create a Spa dedicated to helping people lose weight painlessly.

Dr. Jolliffe aided him in developing the program, most

importantly the nutritional therapy. Larry Paskow became Dr. Jolliffe's faithful student, and today is one of the world's outstanding authorities on nutrition. He has never ceased his studies and research and takes great joy in teaching others to understand the relationship of physical and mental health and vigor to sound nutrition.

But his teachings didn't prevent Stuart, while operating the Spa in New Jersey, from becoming overweight, putting 210 pounds on his five-foot-11-inch body. The weight gain happened rapidly.

"Tension. Frustration," Stuart states succinctly. "I ate six meals a day and didn't even notice I was gaining weight. Then one morning I stepped from the shower and got a good look at myself in a full-length mirror. I didn't like what I saw and right then I put myself on the Harbor Island Spa regime. I continue to eat six meals a day, but they're modest-sized ones, and contain no junk whatsoever. Now when I glimpse myself in the mirror, I like what I see. I'll never be fat again."

Today Stuart weighs 158 pounds.

It usually takes a shock to trigger a decision to reduce.

A 22nd birthday brought Amy to us. Five feet eight inches tall and weighing 198 pounds, Amy had retreated from the world. Refusing to go out, refusing to look for a job, refusing to see friends, Amy stayed in her room except at meal times and immediately thereafter she returned to her room, now armed with cookies and other snacks. But hear Amy, now bubbling and ebullient, tell her own story:

"I checked into the Spa suffering from headaches, arthritis, and a total sense of worthlessness. I went to the Spa with the encouragement of my father, who loves thin women, and against the wishes of my mother, who thought I was wasting my time and their money. With Barbie's sympathetic counsel and clear explanations about nutritional needs, I found no difficulty getting into the program right away. Within eight weeks, I had reduced my weight to 158 pounds. My depression and arthritic pains were gone. And I went out on my first social evening in years. Even enjoyed a cocktail with no feeling of guilt at all. I had counted those calories into my day's allotment. People talked to me. Men asked me to dance. One young man asked me for a date. I felt desirable! It was a miracle. I had a ball."

Since returning to her home in New York State, Amy has found herself a job, is continuing her weight-loss program, and has a new resolve: she is saving to return to college to study nutrition with the goal of developing a career of helping young people who are fat to become normal, healthy, happy young people—and stay that way. Amy periodically returns to the Spa for week-ends "for fun and fresh inspiration."

When people go home, we urge them to be faithful to their diet—six days a week, but on one day out of each seven, we urge they eat as they choose. Otherwise the regime becomes boring and people cheat. Once having started cheating, it's likely to happen with increasing frequency. That seventh no-diet day is a good time to be a guest in someone's home or in a restaurant. If you dine out oftener than that, you don't need to make an issue of your diet but just remember that *your* health is what's important.

To help our Spa guests remember how to eat for the sake of health and joy-in-living, we have, at Harbor Island Spa, created "Ten Commandments for a Thinner, Healthier You"—and a healthy appestat. We suggest that these "Ten Commandments" be affixed to the front or side of your refrigerator—some place where you can see them easily—and often.

Commandment 1: Eat a well-balanced diet, including fats and carbohydrates, limiting your caloric intake to energy output. (1000–1200 calories for women; 1400–1600 for men.)

Commandment 2: Eat slowly, chew thoroughly, and *enjoy* your food.

Commandment 3: Thirty minutes before breakfast, drink 8 ounces of hot water—with or without lemon or prune juice.

Commandment 4: Don't drink cold water immediately before or with meals—for your digestion's sake.

Commandment 5: Do *sip* four to eight glasses of water daily *between* meals—for your digestion's sake.

Commandment 6: Get some exercise daily.

Commandment 7: Don't fast—except possibly for a one-day, one-fruit diet—unless you are under the close and continuing supervision of a physician.

Commandment 8: Ignore your diet one day a week—to avoid monotony and to deter cheating.

Commandment 9: Avoid salt, caffeine, sugar and all "empty" calories.

Commandment 10: For five minutes twice a day, every day, *picture* yourself healthy, slim, happy, vibrant—now!

It will be hard at first, perhaps, to picture yourself as slim, healthy, and exuding joie de vivre, but imagination and *practice* will make it easy very soon, and a reality not too long after that. Tonight, before you fall asleep, relax in your bed, shut your eyes, breathe deeply two or three times and feel your muscles relax. Then draw into your mind a picture of yourself as you would like to be. Do this picturing twice a day for five minutes at a time and, within 30 days, I promise you you will be well on your way to actually being this new, more appealing you. Truly, it is so.

Don't let doubt creep in. If it does, take another deep breath and restore on the screen of your mind the picture of yourself as slim, healthy, vital, attractive. See yourself as being that way *now*. Soon the picture will be the reality.

Andrew Carnegie was one of the great practitioners of visualization. Nightly, he visualized himself discussing his daily affairs—mostly business affairs—with great minds of the centuries. He mentally "talked over" his problems, his decisions, with these great minds and he *listened* to their comments, and invited their suggestions. Andrew Carnegie's habit of visualization is credited by those who know of it as being the true source of his success and wealth.

I don't know who Andrew Carnegie chose as his "mental counselors," but I assume his "board" consisted of men who were rich and powerful—men of his time and earlier. Since health and beauty are your goals, you might like to create for yourself a counseling team of extraordinarily healthy, handsome, and long-lived people, although not all may have started out in life as healthy and handsome. You might, for instance, choose Bernarr Mac-Fadden, who changed from a weakling into an example of the body beautiful; Adonis, the Greek god, whose beauty was so famed we sometimes say "to adonize" when we mean "to beautify"; Venus de Milo, if you are female and large-boned, or Botticelli's Venus if you are female and small-boned; a long-living Ecuadorian to whom you give your favorite Spanish name; a long-living inhabitant of Hunza-land; and may I commend to you Larry and Stuart Paskow? They really care how you feel and look.

As you "counsel" with your "health and beauty board," listen to their health and beauty recommendations, and picture yourself as *one with them*—healthy and beautiful—and soon you will find the will to resist eating more than is good for you. You will find the pounds dropping away. Possibly you may even eat oftener than you do now, but instead of your habits of today, which are putting fat on, you'll find that you are eating to make yourself thin and that, indeed, your hunger has been in your head. As your appestat becomes repaired, you will be thinner, healthier, happier. Man or woman, tall or short, large-boned or small, you will be beautiful. And you will eat well, eat often, and you will enjoy it.

Chapter 2

Handicaps of Fat—Financial, Social, and Emotional

EVERY overweight person is a handicapped person. Recognition of that fact should help prevent obesity—and help motivate the presently obese to do something about their problem. The handicap of overweight usually makes itself felt in every aspect of a person's life—employment, health, fulfillment of emotional/sexual needs.

When seeking a particular job or career appointment, an overweight person can find himself rejected in favor of someone normal-sized because of the job-seeker's self-consciousness about his weight or the potential employer's prejudice against fat people. By law, job applicants are to be treated equally. Fat is not supposed to be a consideration. But in countless cases it is. If you get fat on the job, that's different. You can't be fired for being fat.

Fat can be a handicap in social relationships. Fat can be a handicap in realizing a dream to marry. Fat can be a handicap if marriage does take place. Fat can deter or prevent conception because obese men are more likely to be sterile. Fat can be a handicap in sexual intercourse. And when an overweight woman does become pregnant, she faces special hazards: one being that stillbirths are more frequent among obese mothers.

Overweight is a serious health hazard. Insurance studies show that the mortality rate for the overweight in specific age brackets is much higher than for men and women of normal weight. One insurance study shows that men who were as little as 10 percent overweight had a 16 percent excess mortality over normal men, while men who were as much as 30 percent overweight had a 42 percent excess mortality!

Obese men are more likely to die of heart attacks, cancer, diabetes, digestive diseases, strokes, high blood pressure, and kidney diseases. Surgical procedures take longer because of the layers of fat and stretched tissues with which the surgeon must contend, and anesthesia is more dangerous.

Fat is a financial burden—in everything from the cost of insurance (some companies give the normal-size persons lower rates) to food to clothes. Not only is clothing for the overweight frequently more costly, there is less variety to choose from. As for food bills, fat accumulation and maintenance are costly! Ask anyone who has had a fatso as a house guest for any length of time. A woman carrying 50 excess pounds requires about 200 extra calories daily—or about 8 percent above what food costs would be if her weight were normal.

The obese suffer in relationship to success in work, in social relationships, in their health potential, and, most particularly, they suffer emotionally. Emotional problems are both a result and a cause of obesity.

When people are tense and unhappy they usually respond in one of two ways: they "can't eat" or they eat compulsively. Some thin people eat compulsively too (and rapidly) during periods of extreme stress, but, when the crisis is past, they no longer overeat. Instead, usually, their food consumption drops below normal, the result of that well-functioning appestat that prompts an automatic reduction in food consumption to compensate for the food binge.

According to a Johns Hopkins Medical School study, 75 percent of fat people respond to stress by eating. Stress has many forms and has as many causes as there are people—in the broad view. Every aspect of life carries its potential of stress—from being born, to learning to walk, to learning discipline, from school days to friendships, to love, to personal and professional goals, hobbies, and other interests. Millions, continuously, or even occasionally, disappointed feed their hunger for approval, love, and applause with food.

Researchers have found many fascinating facts about the overweight, among them:

1) Instead of being satisfied with themselves, as many "normal" people are inclined to believe about fat people, they are

plagued by a conviction of inadequacy and ugliness.

2) They have an exceptionally low level of tolerance to frustration.

3) They picture themselves as larger than they really are. (If you are one of them, this is all the more reason for you to practice faithfully picturing yourself, twice daily, morning and evening, as slim and trim.)

4) They often compensate for feelings of inadequacy by aggressive and abrasive behavior.

5) Feelings of unworthiness and hostility may trigger hormonal mechanisms that lead to a craving for food.

While physiological disturbances sometimes are factors in obesity and there is apparent evidence implicating pancreatic, adrenocortical, thyroid, sex, and pituitary hormones in some cases of obesity, there are many who believe that emotions play a part in almost every case of obesity. But fat cannot be excused on the basis of emotions!

Sheer enthusiasm for food, repeated admonitions during childhood to "clean your plate," traditional hunger (that exists among some families who are first- or second-generation immigrants to the bountiful country of America), and traditions of hospitality all may have set up the conditions that led to obesity—and then emotional factors entered in.

Sometimes a tragedy, or series of tragedies, can cause a thin person suddenly to begin eating. Felicia F. is such a person. She was a slim girl, weighing only 110 pounds when she married her childhood sweetheart. He was a Navy flyer; she, a medical student. Within a year she was pregnant, and interrupted her medical studies for a time to devote herself to her young son. Then her husband was killed in Vietnam. She returned to the university, leaving her son much in the care of nurses. During long nighttime hours of study, as she struggled to catch up with her one-time fellow classmates, she ate—initially, she thought, for energy, to compensate for lack of sleep. In less than a year she went from 110 to 150 pounds. Before she completed her medical studies she topped 200 pounds. The wit and humor that had delighted her young husband, her family and friends, turned bitter and caustic, and frequently she erupted into spontaneous rages. As she continued her studies into psychiatry and underwent analysis, she learned neither to reverse her tragedy-provoked angers nor her proclivity for food. She developed diabetes. She began to have problems with her teeth, losing many. Her skin developed innumerable fine lines, a skin that might have been found in a 70- or 80-year-old. Not yet 40, she looks much older. She was brought to Harbor Island Spa one weekend by a friend. In a conversation we had at her first lunch, she revealed she had bought a copy of "The Drinking Man's Diet," but she had not yet read it. It became readily apparent she had little intention of going on a diet, yet she was not without feminine feelings. She apologized because her dress didn't fit well. She asked if I liked the color of her new nail polish. She expressed worry about her health. She announced she had a tumor and said she needed an operation. She feared cancer.

When I asked if she was not concerned about the complications of her overweight in relation to the impending operation, she stated she had no intention of giving up ice cream, cake, and "the other things I like"—regardless of her diabetes or the operation. I gave her a delicious chocolate mousse (you'll find the recipe on page   ). She declared she was "crazy about it," but she said she could not follow our diet because she did not have her own home, lived in hotels, and so would find it difficult to eat pleasurable low-calorie foods. She would drink a quart of "cola" in a single sitting, or eat half a pie or half a cake. She insisted she did not enjoy eating breakfast and that she kept her "weight under control" by eating only once a day.

Her intent on self-destructiveness was deep-seated and intense. We don't have many failures at Harbor Island Spa and I was baffled as to why she bothered to come. She finally explained. She came "as a favor" to her friend. And, I added to myself mentally, to prove to her friend that her weight was "inevitable and unchangeable." She may return. She may decide to lose weight one day, but I doubt it. She is wallowing in unspoken self-pity. Her fat is to demonstrate how much she has suffered from the death of a wonderful husband. She had never had a date since his death yet she talked as if she had to "work and plan" to prevent unwanted overtures from men.

Unspoken hostility to someone, or to some situation or happening, is a frequent trigger for the overeating that leads to obesity. At Harbor Island Spa we found such a baffling situation as the fat man who began to gain weight after his wife went on a diet and reduced from a size 18 to a size 10—the dress size she had worn when she was in her twenties. As we explored why he had gained so much weight, he confessed he had been an incessant eater while sitting in front of the television set at night. Much later in our conversations I learned that he thought his wife had gone on a diet because there was a new man in her life.

In private talks with his wife I found there was no other man.She had been frustrated because her husband was withdrawn from her and she thought if she dieted and became slim again he might take the interest in her that he had had when they were first married. Instead, he became even more withdrawn—hostile, she felt—and gained weight.

It became clear that their real problem was communication. But she at least recognized that her husband was sufficiently concerned about his weight—and her anger about it—that he had come to Harbor Island Spa. When she saw his willingness to cooperate with us, she gave him words of approval. By the time they checked out of the Spa three weeks later, he had lost more than 20 pounds, much of it water, of course, but they were talking to each other. They went home with our diet lists and recipes.

Since then they have returned to us for frequent weekends. His weight continued to go down steadily until it stabilized at 155. From being a tense, unhappy, sexually frustrated couple when they first visited us, today they are radiant with health and happiness. He confessed to me sheepishly on one visit when he was still in his weight-losing period that he was ashamed of himself for having suspected his wife of unfaithfulness. It then developed that he had been unfaithful to her at an earlier period and had been feeling guilty about it.

"I was not meant to be a Romeo," he said, smiling. "I have the best wife in the world and am going to make sure she knows I know it all the rest of our lives." ·

That was more than five years ago. On Palm Sunday in 1976, in New York City, they joined with some 3000 other couples to renew their marriage vows in a church ceremony.

Fat teen-agers have a variety of problems. Mary J., who came to us one summer about four years ago, did so under doctor's orders, but with the full approval of her mother. Mary J.'s story, confessed one afternoon in a storm of tears, was tragic but, sadly, not unique. She started to gain weight the year she was 14 after being raped by her father after he had been fired from his job for alcoholism.

Subsequently her parents were divorced. Mary never told her mother what had happened; never told her doctor. She had been suffering alone with her problem for more than three years. She felt that her life was ruined; that no young man would ever want her as a wife since she was not a virgin. As she talked with me, I was able to make her realize that her tragedy was not unique to her; that the tragedy had not affected her worth as a person; that her father was suffering from a disease that made him incapable of always knowing what he was doing.

Without explaining the problem to her mother or her doctor, we urged that psychological therapy be added to Mary's program. The mother, who had a good position as an executive secretary, was more than willing. On a visit to the Spa to see Mary a few weeks later, she was so pleased with her weight loss and her happier spirits that she proposed that Mary switch colleges and remain with us beyond the summer through the next university year. In that year, Mary became a slim, beautiful young woman, an outstanding student at one of our New Jersey colleges, and highly popular with both sexes. She is now a graduate student, specializing in clinical psychology. She expects to marry one day. Meantime, she has many young-friends and a busy, productive life, living alone in a small apartment near the university and often returning to us at Harbor Island Spa for a weekend for the pleasure of it. Mary is ''family'' to us.

While Mary's mother had no idea about the source of her daughter's problem, her permission and her friendly encouragement helped immeasurably in setting the stage for Mary's transformation from a fat young woman who ate to make herself unattractive to men to a beautiful, happy, confident young woman. Mary's feelings, in the beginning, however, were not at all unlike those expressed by another 17-year-old, who wrote after three months of being on our program:

FORMER FATSO

As you walk into a room
And people stop and stare,
They're looking at your fat
And not your just-done hair.

You look in the mirror
For just one second, of course,
From your eyes comes a tear—
You're built like a horse!

Friends ask you to go bowling
But you're not in the mood;
You see your fat rolling
And gobble down food.

It's your first dance
And kids make fun,
You've got a fat chance
And that's no pun.

When you discover your dress size,
You're really obese—
So you go exercise
Instead of eating a feast.

You're determined not to get discouraged
So you go on a strict diet.
How else could Raquel Welch have emerged?
One look at her body—you wish you could buy it.

Finally, you decide to really abide
By a really and true scarce menu,
You get down teeny and wear a bikini;
Guys whistle, not make fun of you.

One mother called me, saying her daughter would be checking in at the Spa and must be put on 440 calories a day. I told her the lowest diet we had was 600 calories, and I asked how her daughter felt about going on such a stringent diet.

She replied, "It doesn't matter what she thinks. She's obese."

Kathy M., 16, told me: "My parents are constantly after me about my weight at every meal. I get so upset sometimes I refuse to come out of my room at mealtime, but I make up for my frustration by eating after they go to bed."

41

But she didn't want to be fat and had been taking appetite suppressants, water pills, and had tried fasting. Each gave her a temporary weight loss, but as soon as she stopped taking pills or stopped fasting, the weight returned. With our sensible and pleasurable menus, she lost weight. More important, or as important, she kept it off.

A person who would appear to be one of those rare exceptions whose obesity seemingly has no emotional undertones is Harry F., a handsome, highly successful businessman who, at 60 and 60 pounds overweight, already has survived two heart attacks. In social situations he always eats normally—except that his normal social situation centers around luxurious food. He is a member of several wine and food societies. A Marine officer during World War II, after the war, he entered upon his business career with an almost immediate success and, more as a hobby than for any business reason, he became part owner of one of the world's most distinguished restaurants. With a great capacity for friendship and admiration for the arts, his life seemed to offer everything, including, spaced rather far apart, two talented and pretty wives. Both marriages ended in divorce. Since the second divorce, he has had many "dates" but few steady relationships other than deep and steadfast friendships. Periodically he diets, but his taste for food is stronger than his desire to lose weight—the heart attacks notwithstanding. He does not "raid the ice box" or nibble between meals but at mealtime he demands the best, and while he tries, now, to avoid sauces, his fish is broiled or sauteed in butter, baked potatoes are lavished with butter or sour cream, occasionally he succumbs to creamy chocolate mousse or cheese cake or pecan pie, and rarely a meal passes that he does not have wine with it. There are no emotional implications in his overweight, insofar as Harry F. has ever indicated. He attributes his fat to the sheer enjoyment of good food.

A totally different overweight male is Norman P., redheaded and "easily riled." Short, volatile, bright, attractive, he is more than 25 pounds overweight—all of it centered in his midsection. He gets up early—5 o'clock—for no known reason except habit and for a leisurely two-hour breakfast. After a walk with his dog, he's back in time to breakfast with his wife. A midmorning snack at 10 helps carry him through to lunch. A 4 o'clock snack takes him to 6 o'clock supper. By eight, or at the latest nine, he is in bed, sleeping, nudged along by a sturdy nightcap—often bourbon in milk, laced with sugar. He is 52, has been separated from his wife on several occasions. An early retiree, he is bored. Eating is his chief reason-for-being. The sports he still indulges in, though far less often than in the past, aren't sufficient compensation for his near-incessant food intake. He too was a Marine in World War II. He too made a success in business— sufficient to allow him to retire at 48, and he is frank to state that his basic problem is boredom. Creative, he is trying to write a mystery novel and has taken a commonplace job recently simply to protect himself from the handy kitchen with its ever-full stock of delicious food. He has had frequent and serious warnings about his health— open-heart surgery, peptic ulcer, and psoriasis—to name just three grave problems. He has his drinking controlled to prelunch, predinner, prebedtime, but he has not yet braced himself to the fact that he is eating/drinking himself into an early grave, into divorce, and into ever-increasing frustration.

Lacking interests in life, people often resort to food for something to do, and condition their appestats to an overly high level in consequence. This condition is called "psychological bulimia." Another manifestation of psychological bulimia is the fat unmarried woman in whom obesity represents an escape from male attention, with its potential of marriage and duties and responsibilities as wife and mother. Another is the slim bride who, in a few years, becomes grossly fat, a direct, though unconscious, response to finding the attentions from her husband less than she had expected—sometimes because he is overly involved in his work or business, or even because he is busily occupied with women other than his wife. If she discovers her husband is unfaithful, she, by having become fat, subconsciously provides her husband with a reason to forgo sex relations with her. A healthy-minded person would seek a positive solution to the marital problem—by changing herself or the situation, or by accepting it philosophically and making adjustments that are not harmful to her health and emotional well-being.

Similarly, a child who feels unwanted may become a big eater because, subconsciously, food symbolizes security to him. A poorly adjusted adolescent, feeling rejected by his or her peers, can find solace in oral gratification and develop a pattern of overeating as a crutch for an unsatisfied ego. Adults who are hungry for acceptance and recognition, and those whose needs for affection are not adequately met, can try to compensate for these unmet needs by increased food intake.

Anger, hostility, fear, anxiety, even feelings of insecurity can disrupt the proper workings of your appestat and set in motion a pattern of overeating. If you are obese, examine your moods and emotions—your feelings about yourself, your family, your friends (*true* feelings). If your feelings are generally negative, your mind is playing havoc with your appestat and your appestat in turn is demanding food and putting those unwanted pounds on you—unwanted or you would not be reading this book.

Since you have progressed thus far, hopefully it will require only awareness of the direct relationship between negative emotions and fat to make you consciously and conscientiously practice feeling optimistic, and cause you to take a positive view of life. Negativism sets up bad "vibes" for everyone. Everyone around you is a victim, but the biggest victim is you yourself.

When one of our guests, Arthur M., 40, told me of his feelings of being "so ugly," I asked if he related his feelings of "inner ugliness" to a specific picture.

"Yes," he said. "I picture my skin covering an inch of fat—lard—like a well-fattened pig. That picture keeps coming back into my mind, recurring and recurring. When I'm attracted to a woman, I hold back. I see that fat—my gross body—and can't believe any woman would want to speak to me, let alone go out with me."

"Many fat men are very successful with women," I responded. "Why don't you remember that?"

"I *know* that," Mr. M. said, "but I can't believe it. Anyway, every time I see an attractive woman with a fat man I decide he must have something else going for him—wealth, for instance, or power."

"You aren't a poor man," I commented. "You have a good business. You certainly are well able to afford a wife and family."

"I know," he said. "I just can't forget my fat."

Six months later, 25 pounds lighter, Arthur M., who made a practice of coming to the Spa every weekend, started dating one of our other dieting guests. Little more than a year afterwards, when he was nearly 40 pounds lighter and she had reduced from a size 18 to a size 12, they were married at the Spa. That was three years ago. They are frequent visitors with us now, often spending a week or two at a time, and each is a happy, energetic, outgoing person; their weights are stabilized, respectively, at 164 and 130.

"We understand each other," Martha M. told Stuart Paskow and me one evening in "Stuart's Place," when she and her husband were enjoying a cocktail-hour "Barbie Special" (1 ounce vodka, 4 ounces unsweetened cranberry juice over crushed ice).

Her doting husband reached out and took her hand. "She supports me in everything I do," he said. "She's a beautiful cook. We enjoy every mealtime together. And we not only enjoy the taste, we enjoy knowing that the food we eat is good for us—that we're taking care of our bodies and our minds. In my fat days, when the normal office day was through, all I did was go on working. Now, our evenings are filled with activity—things we do together, like go bowling or to the theater or even out dancing, or often we entertain friends at home or go to friends' homes."

"We've even joined a political club," Martha said, "and we've become involved in a city beautification program."

"And how's your business, Arthur?," Stuart asked.

"That's the astonishing part," he answered. "It's better than it ever was—more than a third again what it used to be—both sales and profits."

"That's because you're so brilliant and charming and helpful to your customers," Martha said, with a teasing smile, but meaning it. "You know," she said, turning to Stuart and me, "people seek Arthur out, to be with him. His unfailing interest in other people makes him the 'center of attention' at every party."

Arthur laughed. "It's funny," he said, "how easy it is to make friends. All one needs to do is demonstrate that you truly are interested—that you're sincere. It's a fact I wish every fat person knew, but I didn't discover it until I lost weight."

"As I recall," Stuart remarked, "your business involves a lot of stress."

"Sure," Arthur responded, "but now I can handle it. When I was fat, my response was to eat rather than examine how I might solve the problem. Now solving the problem is fun, and I never think of eating. Stress sure isn't reduced by eating; only aggravated."

Some—many—fat people have gone to psychiatrists about their weight, but psychiatry has not been notably successful in

45

producing "cures." Talking out problems is good for everyone, but, unless the counsel is combined with a nutritional program designed to create a healthy internal environment along with weight loss, the expenditure of time and money is not likely to achieve permanent weight loss.

An emotional problem that afflicts most fat people is the belief that "normal" people view their fat as evidence of greedy self-indulgence, and, to a large extent, "normal" people do. It is a sad fact that the general population ignores the uniqueness of the individual and demands conformity—at least of shape.

Most fat people have a fear of walking into a room filled with people. They are afflicted by such overbearing fears as that their clothes are too tight and showing all the bulges of their ugly bodies, or that someone thin is staring at them—scornfully or, just as bad, pityingly.

When they visit hotels that are on the "family plan," with set meal hours, just before meal time they often wait in front of the dining room so that they can be first in and first out, or order room service so that no one can see them eat. They constantly worry about what people are saying about them, or thinking about them. They worry about going to the beach or getting up on the dance floor. They have the feeling everyone else gets what he wants: jobs, compliments, friends, dates, love.

All of this changes for them at the Spa. It's amazing how fast they can change from wary, distrustful, unhappy to appreciative, open, even enthusiastic once they know someone cares and is really out to help them without criticism, without blame, without ridicule. In "The Truth About Weight Control," Dr. Neil Solomon describes what Dr. Arthur Kornhaber, a psychiatrist, calls the "Stuffing Syndrome." Dr. Kornhaber says the primary symptoms are constant overeating, depression, and withdrawal. He likened overeating, without regard for hunger or the effect on the body, and late-night "stuffing" to an animal preparing to go into hibernation.

In the "Stuffing Syndrome" Dr. Kornhaber finds early signs of a severe depression. It may also be, he suggests, a substitute for sexual activity, which leads to further withdrawal, worsened by feelings of guilt that in turn lead to further regression.

Very few of the visitors to Harbor Island Spa are under

psychiatric care, but we have found that those who are generally lose weight at the same rate as do our other obese guests.

Motivation is a basic key to losing weight. Ultimately, it is the unique makeup of the individual that determines how long it will require to achieve and maintain ideal weight. When the motivation can be reinforced and stimulated by psychiatric counsel, that is most desirable. So we make informal counseling a basic activity at Harbor Island Spa—though not all of our guests recognize it as that. As far as the majority are concerned we may just be "having a conversation." We like it that way. When I can stimulate a guest into having a bit more confidence, a bit more belief that weight loss is an achievable goal, I'm thrilled. I feel as if I were walking on air, for I know then that the goal of weight loss is likely to be realized.

While emotions play a part in the majority of cases, it would be wrong to ignore the physiological factors that exist in every case. It is essential that psychological and physiological conditions be taken into consideration simultaneously. A program of positive thinking—a conscious program—plus exercise, plus diet reform are the three foundation stones on which you must create the new, slimmer, more vibrant, healthier, happier you.

Chapter 3

Dangers of Fasts, Fads, and Crash Diets

THE person suffering from overweight can easily be tempted by those simple-sounding quick-loss diets such as the "rice diet," the "grapefruit diet," the low-carbohydrate "drinking man's diet," and others.

Some years ago an acquaintance went on a high-fat diet, telling all her friends—anyone who would listen—that there were no calories in fat, and she could eat all the fat she wanted and get thin. A few months later she had lost about 30 pounds, inclusive of her gall bladder. In a few more months all 30 pounds were back, and a few more too. But not her gall bladder.

Talking about diets, going on diets is a great American pastime. But for the obese, who suffer mental anguish and, often, physical discomfort, there is nothing funny about the cracks about fat that TV and nightclub comedians like to indulge in, and when a new Messiah comes along with a "fast, sure way to lose weight," thousands listen.

Americans are the fattest people on earth. We are also among the sickest, with many of those diseases directly related to overweight, and some to trying to lose weight too fast.

It is almost impossible for you to maintain healthy low weight on a "fad" diet. First of all, you need well-balanced dietary guidelines by which to revise your eating habits. Second, limitation of your intake of "essential nutrients" tends to throw your system out of kilter and cause deep-seated nutritional problems.

For this reason, many people lose weight and then gain it back because, by the time they resume regular eating, their metabolic system has ceased to behave normally and their bodies may be storing considerable fat simply because their food is not being used or burned up properly.

48

Low-Carbohydrate Diet:

Going on a low-carbohydrate diet will cause a drop in weight—provided you don't eat or drink too many calories. Medical research shows that when you drastically reduce your carbohydrate intake, your body dumps salt and water, and water, of course, represents a large percentage of the body's total weight.

But a no-carbohydrate, or very low-carbohydrate, diet, with no restrictions on intake of fats and proteins can do grave damage to the nervous system, heart, and brain.

There are people whose bodies demand more carbohydrates than what is considered the minimum requirement for the average person. Such people may develop hypoglycemia if they do not have adequate carbohydrates in their diet. The hypoglycemic, or hypoglycemic-prone, needs extra carbohydrates for nourishment of his brain and the retina of his eyes. Because such a person has a lower concentration of glucose or of sugar in the circulating blood, his brain is not properly nourished, nor is the retina of the eye. Thus hypoglycemics often complain that their mental efficiency is slowed down.

Too many carbohydrates is equally dangerous. Too many carbohydrates would cause the pancreas to secrete more insulin, which would burn up sugar at such a rate that the blood sugar would fall to a dangerous level. Thus the physician should determine just how much carbohydrate the hypoglycemic should have in his diet.

Many people who restrict their carbohydrates experience fatigue caused by various metabolic changes such as excessive loss of body fluids, of sodium and minerals, ketosis, and loss of nitrogen. Certain researchers believe the result may also be a breakdown of body protein tissue (essentially muscle) and bone.

High-Protein Diet:

Our Harbor Island Spa diets include considerable primary protein, but never an excessive amount. In the fad high-protein diet, the dieter is directed to eat nothing, or practically nothing, except meat, cheese, fish, and eggs. The human body has only limited storage for protein, so any excessive protein will be converted into fat or, through a process know as gluconeogenesis, into sugar. Anyone with a tendency towards gout, arthritis, diabetes, or any medical problem in which urea nitrogen, ketone bodies, or electrolyte balance are poorly handled, should avoid a high-protein diet. A high-protein diet can cause an obese person to develop a kidney infection or kidney malfunction. If a person with an existing kidney infection or malfunction were to go on a high-protein diet, the dieter would retain urea and the result would be coma and even death. The likelihood is remote, it's true, but the basic fact still remains—the human body requires a rounded diet.

High-Fat Diet:

Overabundance of fat in the diet can cause diarrhea, which will cause weight loss but which will also cause a loss of essential vitamins, minerals, and cofactors, compounds essential for functioning of the enzymes. Loss of fluid is also a danger. Serious dehydration means the body cells are being depleted of the fluids they need for survival. Electrolytes, such as magnesium, potassium, and sodium, are lost and, if they cannot be replaced quickly, this condition too can cause coma and death.

Low-Fat Diet:

Diets should be low in fat, but some fat is essential. Fats provide us with our most concentrated form of energy and combine with phosphorus to form part of every cell. Fats are particularly concentrated in brain and nerve tissues. The kidneys, heart, and liver are supported by small layers of fat. Under your skin there is a padding of fat that cushions the nerves and muscles and helps to protect the body from sudden changes in temperature. The emaciated who do not have this cushioning of fat suffer from nervousness and fatigue, as well as the appearance of premature aging, and can develop skin rashes and kidney disorders.

Diets too low in fat can cause dry skin and scalp and decreased lubrication of the joints among other problems.

Even a reducing diet should contain 30 to 33 percent fat.

One-Dimensional Diets:

Some medical doctors recommend one-dimensional diets for quick weight loss; but ordinarily only for a week or two, in which time the obese may lose five to 15 or more pounds. Among such diets, approved by certain doctors for HEALTHY INDIVIDUALS, are:

●Bananas and skim milk, alternating one banana and one glass

50

of milk over nine periods during the day for a total of 900 calories.

●All-vegetable diet, eating as many vegetables as you wish up to six meals daily.

●Cottage cheese and grapefruit diet or cottage cheese and melon for a total of six meals daily.

●Buttermilk only—six glasses over the course of a day.

●Baked potato and buttermilk—one baked potato, with skin, daily, together with six glasses of buttermilk.

●Twelve slices of bread daily—plus whatever else you want to eat.

●Meat, fish, or poultry only, together with plenty of water.

●Grapes only, or apples only—all you wish to eat.

At Harbor Island Spa, we recommend against such drastic diets. While some claim they have no adverse effects, if is possible that unfortunate results may show up later. In any event, we urge you not to try a bizarre diet on your own without a doctor's supervision, or, if you are insistent upon doing it without supervision, please, not for more than a day or two at the most.

Though various doctors contend their patients suffer no ill effects, except possibly light-headedness, if they stay on any of these one-dimensional diets a few weeks or even a few months, I must caution you. These diets are dangerous, except possibly the 12-slices-of-bread-daily, providing you eat a variety of food along with the bread, such as fresh fruits and vegetables, protein, and some fat.

While most people are likely to be so bored with one-dimensional dieting that they won't remain on it long enough to bring their body to any danger point, the fact is that, even when the weight comes off, unless the quick "fad" is followed promptly by a nutritionally sound, low-calorie diet, the fat will return. Permanent weight loss requires creation of a healthy internal environment, and that can be accomplished only when you eat a well-balanced diet including protein, fats, carbohydrates, vitamins, minerals, and water.

The Harbor Island Spa diets in this book contain a high portion of protein to carbohydrates but they are not devoid of carbohydrates nor are they lacking in any other nutritional essential. They are balanced diets.

Chapter 4

Sound Nutrition: Key to a Healthy Appestat and Healthy Old Age

CERTAIN scientists have claimed that if they had a hundred billion dollars they could discover how people could live to 120 years and stay in good health all of the time. One of the first things they would have to do, they say, is find a way to prevent hardening of the arteries, which, in too many Americans, begins early. This pervasive "American disease" has been found to exist even in children—and in thousands of soldiers in Vietnam.

A basic factor in hardening of the arteries is high blood pressure. Our blood pressure is affected by psychological and physiological factors, and it can be reduced by what we eat, how much we eat, and how we eat it, as well as by our mental attitudes. A high cholesterol count is also implicated in hardening of the arteries. High blood pressure and a high cholesterol count are found in the majority of the obese, so losing weight can mean a big step forward to a healthy old age. This is without further burdening taxpayers with finding that hundred billion dollars to discover how we can grow old healthily.

It isn't enough simply to want to lose weight. Choose a bigger, more important goal: decide that you will be healthy and happy as well as slim.

To be healthy you must eat—and well. You must really enjoy your food, and with the recipes you find in this book I am confident you will.

The objective of our method is to eliminate worry about weight by establishing, through sound nutrition, an internal environment conducive to the re-creation of a healthy appestat. That way, in time, the appestat functions properly, the caloric intake vs. caloric output becomes automatic, and a person routinely stays at his ideal weight.

When your appestat functions properly, you will find you automatically eat more when you are expending extra energy—when you play tennis all day or when you are recuperating from an illness or when you are in your teen and pre-teen years and need extra calories for your body's growth. When your energy expenditure is less, your appetite automatically lessens. If you happen to overindulge at one meal, you eat less automatically at the next, or you take a good, long, brisk walk to get rid of that feeling of oversatiety.

The diets in this book are designed to produce weight loss while eating to the point of satisfaction and, most importantly, to create that healthy environment for the appestat.

The appestat is located in the hypothalamus, which is in the brain at the base of the skull near the pituitary gland. In this region of the brain are other automatic regulating centers, such as for body temperature, sleep, and water balances. A few rare diseases can damage the appestat, such as a tumor of the pituitary gland and encephalitis (sleeping sickness) with resulting bulimia (appetite in excess of the body's needs). Bulimia leads to obesity. A pancreatic tumor, secreting large amounts of insulin, may also cause a form of bulimia; and overtreatment of diabetes with insulin, if continued long enough, may condition the appestat to a higher-than-necessary level of food intake, making it difficult for the diabetic to be satisfied with less than an excessive amount of food.

Appestat function can be disrupted by negative emotions too, such as hostility, insecurity, anxiety, and so forth—a very good reason for the obese (for everyone) to conscientiously practice feelings of optimism.

An extremely low basal metabolism can cause the appestat to work at a level lower than normal for the energy output. But organic conditions leading to a lower-than-normal or higher-than-normal appestatic level are so rare medical science generally has concluded that such causes are far too infrequent to account for the high obesity rate in the United States.

While it's difficult to obtain precise figures, various research studies have brought the conclusion that, of the 215 million in the United States, some 75 to 79 percent are overweight. One national study states nearly one-fifth of children are overweight by the time they graduate from high school!

Women, over the past 20 years, have been decreasing in average weight, a direct result undoubtly of growing "fashion consciousness," whereas men, in the same period, have been gaining in weight. This is one basic reason why you should not use "average" weights to decide what your "best" weight should be. Women are most likely to gain weight at two periods of life: when pregnant and after menopause; while men gain between ages 25 and 40 but show their greatest acceleration of weight after 40.

It's increasingly popular to blame overweight on psychological factors, but the diagnosis of psychological bulimia is frequently unjustified. There are probably just as many thin people with unresolved emotional problems as there are obese ones. Despite innumerable evidences of psychological overeating, that is not the basic cause of obesity. To blame obesity on psychological problems is just as bad for the obese as to attribute obesity to "glands" or "heredity." Why? Because such diagnoses tend to make the obese person feel he is not responsible for his obesity and that he can't do anything about it personally. To lose weight, a person must focus on the simple fact:

If you eat less, you'll lose weight.

To be slim and healthy—and to produce that essential healthy environment for the appestat—a person must keep this additional fact in mind:

If you eat a well-balanced diet, you will be healthy, and your appestat will be too—in time.

The body requires six "key nutrients": protein, carbohydrates, fats, vitamins, minerals, and water.

These combine to:

1) Build and repair body tissue, including that in the brain.
2) Provide heat and energy.
3) Maintain the regulatory system.

Nutritional imbalances can be caused by too much of any one of the "key nutrients."

To achieve your ideal weight, you should also review your daily pattern of activities. Some people gain weight on a caloric intake that would cause others to lose weight. The difference is due to a difference in activity. Most teen-agers truly do seem to have a "bottomless pit" when it comes to eating and yet remain slim and trim. That is because their energy output is high. When a person's energy output is low, the food input should be low too. But that does not mean restricting one's meals to one or two a day. Stuart Paskow, remember, maintains his ideal weight while eating six meals a day—modest-sized ones. How many calories of food you eat should be equated to your activity pattern. If you aren't very active and take frequent rest periods, you should eat less than a person who is going steadily all day long.

Fat people often tell me they "eat hardly anything." And they really believe it. That's because repeated overeating has set the appestat at a level so high satisfaction can not be obtained at a normal level of food intake. When the appestat is thus conditioned, a person is not conscious of overeating and his appestat isn't going to be returned to normal within a few days after, probably, years of being at an elevated level. It will be brought down slowly and, when it is restored to a normal level, a smaller intake of food will satisfy. When a person cheats and breaks his diet, he is contributing to keeping his appestat high. When a person feels uncomfortable during the first days of being on a highly reduced caloric intake—down, say, from 3000 to 1000 calories a day—his discomfort reflects the appestat's protest against a change of its level.

(Since the words "calorie" and "caloric" are used here frequently, it is appropriate to explain them more fully. Technically, a calorie is the quantity of energy [heat] needed to raise the temperature of 2.2 pounds of water one degree centigrade. In physiology that calorie is used to express the fuel or energy value of food and, sometimes, the quantity of food capable of producing such an amount of energy.)

Elevated appestats can have such varied causes as "raiding the ice box," insatiable nibbling, continual tasting—a job hazard of many professional and good home cooks—and overuse of alcohol. When the alcoholic is fat, it means the appestat has been elevated. But most of us also know very thin alcoholics, a result of a perfectly functioning appestat so that the imbiber's appetite for food diminishes to compensate for the overindulgence in alcohol. However, the resulting insufficient intake of all the "key nutrients" almost inevitably produces a deficiency disease.

Diets must be adapted to the individual. The phrase "well-balanced diet" is taken by many to mean a "standard" diet, standard quantities, but this is wrong. Everyone needs a "well-balanced diet" but the ways to achieve it are almost limitless. A good rule to follow is to have as much variety in your food intake as possible so that you can be sure you are getting sufficient of the six key nutrients your good health requires.

You can follow any of the menus contained in this book, but as general rules your diet should:

1. Contain sufficient high-value protein to prevent body tissues (muscles and organ tissues) from being utilized for protein. (Symptoms of protein depletion include nervousness, a sense of fatigue with inadequate cause, and general weakness.)

2. Contain sufficient carbohydrates to prevent acidosis (from too rapid burning of fat) or lipemia (from too much fat being dispersed into the blood).

3. Get slightly less than one-third of its calories from fat.

4. Contain adequate minerals, vitamins, and water.

5. Contain sufficient fiber to encourage optimum functioning of the elimination system.

Dr. Jolliffe taught that the high consumption of fat by Americans was our most serious nutritional error. We eat more fat per person than any other people, obtaining, on an average, almost half our calories from fat. This is a fact Dr. Jolliffe and other medical practitioners equate with our high prevalence of atherosclerosis, a condition that all too frequently leads to coronary heart disease. If you aren't inclined to give up fat because you are convinced you need not worry about heart disease, just remember this: fat slows down the rate at which carbohydrates and protein are digested.

High-value protein is found in poultry, fish, meat, eggs, shellfish, milk, milk products, and soybeans, but your body requires less than you may believe: only about one gram per day for each two pounds of your *ideal* body weight. If you now weigh 200 pounds but your ideal weight is 150 pounds, you need less than three ounces of protein per day, preferably spread over three meals. Contrast that with the American habit of equating a one-pound steak to a superior meal! To help make the picture clearer: one pound of raw meat will produce, when cooked, approximately three four-ounce servings or two six-ounce servings.

Carbohydrates are contained in cereals, bread, and many fruits and vegetables, all of which are good for you, but if you hunger for cake, please restrict yourself to angel food—easy to digest and low in carbohydrates.

Raw fruits and vegetables are essential. You require them for their vitamins, minerals, and enzymes. They can help prevent build-up of cholesterol. Fruits and vegetables are essential insurance for getting the key nutrients your body requires. They are high in cellulose, beneficial in the prevention of ordinary constipation. Since few eat as many raw fruits and vegetables as they should, and the most careful cooking produces loss of vitamins, minerals, and enzymes, we also recommend, at Harbor Island Spa, vitamin capsules to contribute to optimum health.

It's beneficial to familiarize yourself with the calorie count of standard portions of common foods. Until the caloric values of your favorite foods are firmly fixed in your mind, it's practical to refer to a calorie-carbohydrate "counter" or little book. There are several available at low cost, and the United States Department of Agriculture issues handbooks on the nutritive value and caloric content of foods.

Larry Paskow teaches that breakfast is the most important meal of the day and recommends that we gain most of our day's high-value protein at breakfast. This is a radical departure from the affluent-society routine of dinner being the biggest meal of the day (sometimes with high-value protein in several courses, such as pate or seafood as an appetizer, followed by a fish, poultry, or meat course; and, on gala or formal occasions, a protein appetizer followed by fish followed by a meat course).

Larry Paskow likes to say, "For optimum health, eat breakfast like a king, lunch like a prince, and dinner like a pauper."

While that is what Larry Paskow says, and follows, at the Spa, in this book you'll find that our menus conform more to our dietary traditions, with more elaborate meals at lunch and dinner. These menus always include desserts—made without sugar and with little or no fat. A dessert performs three important functions:

1) keeps people from feeling deprived;
2) satisfies our national sweet tooth;
3) provides a particular feeling of dietary satisfaction.

If you want to switch around our breakfast and dinner menus, go ahead and do it. It's the total caloric intake and nutritional balance that's important.

A high-protein breakfast—that might mean a soft-boiled egg, or a small portion of lean beef, or cottage cheese—raises the blood sugar more slowly than a high-carbohydrate breakfast. Thus the sugar level, with protein, stays higher longer so that the midmorning slump is avoided, together with that craving for a snack that millions of Americans satisfy with "coffee and Danish," a pernicious habit that is a Number One enemy for a health-seeking person.

Any extended self-denial during the first half of the day seldom leads to decreased overall caloric intake. When a person goes without breakfast, he is likely to eat a large lunch, a large dinner, and even have a bedtime snack.

A good reducing diet should lay the foundation for a sensible diet that a person can follow indefinitely—and enjoy. Since satiety value is very important to avoidance of any sense of hunger, we include some protein in each meal. Our diets are low in calories, comparatively high in protein, and low in carbohydrates and fat. If we gave our dieters nothing but beverages, fruits, and vegetables, they would lose weight but they would feel unsatisfied. We normally include a low-calorie snack between 3 and 5 o'clock—fruit or vegetable juice, or half a grapefruit—and for hypoglycemics, and anyone who desires it, a bedtime snack. This might be diet jello and/or a hot beverage. But the food consumed in these snack periods must be counted in the total day's caloric allowance.

At the Spa we approach each person as an individual with an individual weight problem. Our first concern is to make each person feel at ease about his weight problem and talk openly about it. Each person is encouraged to set an achievable weight-loss goal, and that is what I urge you, the reader, to do. Whether you are 10 or 100 pounds overweight, write down the weight you desire to be. Remember that your ideal weight will be affected by your bone structure. A heavy-boned person naturally should weigh more than a small-boned person of the same height.

Variation of 5 to 10 percent over or under the "ideal" weight for height and bone structure are of no real significance in terms of health. But an individual who weighs 10 to 20 percent more than the theoretical norm for his bone structure must be classed as overweight, and anyone who is 20 percent or more above the ideal must be termed obese.

Once you have selected your weight goal, there is much work to be done. Problems such as hunger will arise, and each must find a method to cope with it—free food snacks and the like. (Free foods are those that are virtually calorie-free, such as mushrooms, celery, cauliflower, cabbage, cucumber, sauerkraut, zucchini [delicious raw or steamed], lettuce, and gelatin—that product that does so much good for our teeth, nails, and bones and can turn fruits and vegetables into delightful desserts and salads).

It is essential that you recognize there is a large difference between "hunger" and "appetite."

The appestat controls the feeling of hunger but it does not control the kinds of foods you appease it with. Once you know what's "good" and what's "bad" for you, you can satisfy this *feeling* of hunger accordingly, and in time your appestat will less and less frequently trigger a feeling of hunger.

Let me cite an example. Suppose you are the mother of a 10-year-old who comes home from school announcing he's hungry. You offer an apple. He demands ice cream. If he were hungry, he would accept the apple. The demand for ice cream represents appetite, not hunger.

Hunger is the compeling drive to eat without regard for taste or kind. The compelling drive to eat can be controlled, however, and it's done by eating slowly. The simple trick we teach at the Spa is this: Take a mouthful of food. Now put your fork or spoon down on your plate while, savoring every bit, you slowly chew and swallow. Now you are ready for another fork or spoonful. This procedure will teach you to enjoy your food more, as well as teach you to eat slowly and encourage you to eat less.

When you eat at a quickened pace, various problems arise. First, you eat more than you would if you ate slowly. Second, your stomach develops gas from taking in air along with the food. When the gas pockets break up in your system in an hour or so, you feel hungry and are inclined to eat again. Though your body does not need any food, your appestat has been triggered into saying, "Feed me!"

As part of our educational program at the Spa, we point out that body surpluses are stored in layers of fat. To lose weight, part of this body fat must be used for energy in place of ingested food.

And we urge our dieters to ignore the scales except once a week, and we teach that a tape measure is just as important in measuring loss. We don't weigh or measure oftener than once a week so you won't become discouraged if a particular day does not show a loss—or if it happens to show a slight gain.

Measurements of the chest, midarm, and thigh, waist and hips are important to check at the start of your program to lose weight through eating, and should be checked each week thereafter until you achieve your ideal weight and shape. Often in checking your measurements, you'll find that one or more of these measurements show a change even though the scales may not show a change at all.

But don't allow yourself, in the beginning, to be discouraged by your tape measure either. At first the fat in the tissues may be replaced by water so that your measurements do not show a loss. Don't then resort to diuretics. They have no place in a weight-loss program unless specifically prescribed and supervised by your physician. But eat freely of foods that prevent or reduce water retention, such as beets, potatoes, leafy green vegetables; whole-grain cereals, including wheat and rice; milk and milk products; bananas, cabbage, liver, carrots, egg yolks, and beans, particularly soybeans; and put avocados on your diet too.

The concept of food as fuel that we were taught in elementary school is much too simplistic. Food is much more than fuel, though it is that too, of course. In order to eat to grow thin and create that healthy environment for our appestat, we must learn to appreciate food as far more complex and important than simple energy. We must recognize that what we eat affects how we feel, how we look, how we think, and every element within our bodies.

Chapter 5

Water, Salt, and Caffeine: Benefits and Dangers

WATER, one of the six key elements required for health, in many ways is more important than any other single element. A person can survive weeks without food, using up the body's own tissues for nourishment, but death can result in as short a time as seven to 10 days if one does not have water. Only oxygen is more essential to life.

Few people drink as much water as they should, and most drink it incorrectly. Water, generally, is gulped, particularly if one is very thirsty. Water should be sipped slowly. That way it best benefits the body, just as food, when thoroughly chewed, benefits the body, whereas inadequately chewed food can cause gas and other problems.

Ice water with meals is a bad American habit. So is iced tea, iced coffee, and other cold drinks. Why? A simple reason. Cold water lowers the body temperature, and unless your temperature is at 98.6 degrees, you don't metabolize food properly.

We stress education at Harbor Island Spa. When people learn how the body functions they are more likely to change their bad eating habits for good ones. One of the basic goals is to take the mystique out of good health and replace it with information.

We urge you not to drink coffee, no matter what your age (though we will serve it, if you want it). The medical profession warns us about the dangers of smoking cigarettes. In time, I believe, they may get around to the research that will prove conclusively that caffeine, too, is bad for you, particularly after you reach 40 years of age. For the obese, coffee should be avoided for one reason above all: it stimulates the appetite. And for a great many persons it causes indigestion, as well as other less readily noticeable effects. As a drug, caffeine is useful for one purpose—for stimulating the liver when used in the form of a coffee enema.

At Harbor Island Spa we serve decaffeinated coffee—not Sanka—and we don't serve artificial cream. Preservatives are not what your body needs, particularly not when you are on a diet where every calorie should count for your benefit.

As part of our educational program, we point out that many fat people never lay down knife and fork or spoon when eating. They have these utensils always at the ready, to push in more food—usually before the previous forkful has left their mouths. Result: fat people rarely chew food properly. The more carefully and slowly you chew your food, the better it is digested, the more good it does your body, the more satisfied you feel so that you are inclined to eat less and thereby consume fewer calories.

Food goes from your mouth down your throat and esophagus into the upper stomach. There little hairy substances break up the food into small particles. This upper stomach of ours burns up—metabolizes—food at 98.6 degrees. When you take a cold drink at meal time—water, iced tea, iced coffee, highball, or soft drink—you reduce the body temperature about one-tenth of one degree. You think that is too little to matter? Not true!

When you don't burn your food properly, instead of its being broken into small particles so that the nutrients are readily absorbed and the wastes pass from the body normally, the food remains in larger particles and very often lodges in different areas of your upper and lower intestine. Frequent result: indigestion.

It is to hasten the rise in temperature that we recommend that you drink hot water or hot water and lemon juice or hot water and prune juice on arising. When you get up in the morning after a night's sleep, your temperature is about 98.2 degrees. It takes 15 to 30 minutes of walking around for it to rise to normal level. When you drink hot water you warm the digestive juices to the proper temperature so that the breakfast you eat can be utilized properly and efficiently.

Lemon juice in hot water is particularly beneficial because the citric acid aids digestion. We even suggest you drink a glass of hot water about 30 minutes before each meal, preferably with lemon juice, so that the food you eat later will do you most good.

While we urge you not to drink cold water with your meals, for your digestion's sake, we urge you to drink water between meals so as to aid your digestion. This is not a contradiction. The body requires water. While most vegetables contain a lot of water, much of this is lost in cooking and the body needs to ingest a minimum of 32 ounces a day—sipped, not gulped!

Water promotes the flow of gastric juices and dilutes the food intake.

The reasons to restrict your salt intake, or to avoid salt altogether, are many. For persons with certain diseases or with tendencies toward those diseases, salt should be completely eschewed, and extra zest for the foods you eat should be obtained from lemon, garlic, and other herbs and spices. (The Harbor Island Spa cookbook that is Chapter 13 contains some specific suggestions.)

Excessive salt consumption causes you to retain body fluids, which will make it difficult for you to register weight loss or can even cause a weight gain. For a person with a heart condition, retention of fluids could produce a pulmonary edema—fluid in the lungs, an emergency situation. Hypoglycemics should severely restrict their salt intake because excessive salt consumption causes loss of blood potassium, which in turn leads to a drop in blood sugar. Some women register large weight gains before their periods, the result of excessive salt consumption causing water retention and thereby triggering excessive excretion of a hormone, aldosterone, by the adrenal glands. This hormone causes salt to be retained and potassium lost.

Excessive fluid is not controlled by restricting water consumption but by restricting salt. Restricting your use of table salt should not result in electrolyte depletion because all natural foods contain a certain amount of salt. You will always find salt on the table at Harbor Island Spa, but we caution you in its use and urge you always, wherever you are, to taste your food before you salt it.

Mary J., a pretty young woman of 23, weighed 175 pounds when she came to the Spa. Her legs were badly swollen, even beyond what was normal for her excessive weight, and she had a tingling sensation in her toes and fingers. In my routine investigation of her normal food and drug intake, I learned she had been taking diuretics for many months. When our doctor examined her, he quickly ordered a series of laboratory tests. These showed that she was deficient in potassium, a situation directly attributable to the fact that she had been using an excessive amount of salt on her food. On our low-calorie, well-balanced diet, combined with low salt intake, she lost 30 pounds within the three months she stayed at the Spa; her legs were normal and all sense of ''tingling'' had long since left her fingers and toes. Upon her return home she continued to lose until she stabilized her weight at 115 pounds. She is married now, has one child, and leads an active life.

''Losing weight gave me a whole new life,'' Mary told me when she invited me to her wedding.

Chapter 6

Truths and Fallacies

THERE are many misconceptions about the causes of fat and the ways to lose weight: and even more about food and our nutritional needs. To name a few:

1. Some people remain fat no matter how little they eat, the result of a defect in their basal metabolism.
   False.
   Medical investigation shows that the overweight have no defect in their basal metabolism that can account for their obesity.
2. Malfunctioning of the endocrine glands causes obesity.
   False.
   While some physicians subscribe to this theory, medical research has not been able to show that the overweight generally have any disorder of the endocrine glands to account for their fat. The endocrine glands in part control the distribution of fat but do not control the total amount of fat.
3. Fat people don't use up the same energy that thin people do.
   False.
   Medical experiments have not been able to produce a fat person who uses less energy than otherwise normal people for equal activity. Instead, research shows that the obese expend more energy than normal people because they have a lessened mechanical efficiency. The obese expend more energy than the thin even when lying down.
4. People lose weight when they eat only one meal per day.
   True—sometimes; false—more often.
   For most people, the long period of fasting creates such a hunger they consume more calories at the single meal than they

would have if spaced over three or more rationally planned meals. Research demonstrates that health is improved when meals are spread over the entire day. Breakfast is needed after the night's fast to produce optimum energy in the morning. Lunch provides the energy to carry a person through the afternoon without overfatigue—or any sense of fatigue.

5. Eggs and bananas are hard to digest.

False—generally.

Eggs are slightly more digestible cooked than raw. Soft-cooked eggs are highly digestible. All eggs, including hard-cooked eggs, should be cooked over low heat—whether boiled, fried, poached or scrambled.

Bananas often are eaten unripe. They are ripe when the skins have brown spots. When ripe, bananas are well digested even by a small child. They leave the body slowly and are a superior source of potassium. On a reducing diet, or if hypoglycemic, eat only half a large, or no more than one small banana per day.

6. Fish are brain food.

True—as are countless other foods.

Fish provides phosphorus-containing compounds strengthening to the nerves. But meat, poultry, eggs, and milk also contain phosphorus. The brain as other muscles and tissues—requires a nutritionally balanced diet.

7. Raisins and nuts are required for iron.

False.

Raisins and nuts both contain iron but so do many other foods. Our choices are so many we can easily eliminate any one food from our diet without any harm, providing, of course, we include in our diet comparable foods that together provide the six key nutrients.

8. Many people eat because they are hungry for acceptance and recognition and love.

True.

For such people to lose weight, they must sever the connection between emotions and food.

9. Obesity places added burdens on the heart, circulatory system, liver, and gall bladder.

True.

10. Overweight produces an added risk in surgery.

True.

11. Obesity is a predisposing factor in diabetes, arthritis, gout, and foot troubles.

True.

12. Fat people are jolly.

False—generally.

Some fat people may be jolly, but I do not personally know one.

13. There is a thin body imprisoned within every fat body.

True.

The important thing is to free the thin body from its fat prison slowly so that the skin has a chance to readjust to a smaller circumference; so that a person doesn't become overfatigued from consumption of too little food for the rate of activity; so that the body won't be deprived of the elements essential to good health. Time, patience, and a change of habits and attitude are required for an easy break from the fat prison.

14. Each 10-pound weight loss represents, for women, a decrease in one size of clothing.

True—ordinarily.

15. Fat people regularly describe social occasions in terms of food.

True—sadly.

Food should be an accessory to a social gathering, not the reason for it, unless it's a meeting of a gourmet society.

16. Fat children get that way because, as babies, they were fed too much.

True—ordinarily.

Medical research shows that most fat babies have mothers who ate too much when they were pregnant. Best solution: do not keep candies or cakes or fattening foods around the house. Keep healthy snacks—raw cauliflower, carrot sticks, radishes, cucumbers, and/or fruit—readily available, most particularly when a child comes home from school.

17. Eating scraps left over from the dinner table is "thrifty."

False.

It's thrifty to devise ways to use leftovers for a "second meal" or to feed the leftovers to the family dog or cat. To eat scraps after an adequate-to-good meal is simply fattening.

18. The obese have a shorter life expectancy.

67

True.

19. It's normal for people to gain weight as they grow older.
   False.

People gain weight because they reduce their activities but do not reduce their food consumption—or even increase it. One should weigh *less* at 60 than at 35.

20. Our vitamin and mineral requirements are two major reasons we need food.
   True.

21. The amount of nutrients found in food can vary widely.
   True.

22. Men lose weight faster than women.
   True—ordinarily.

23. You don't have to be anti-social while dieting.
   True.

But you must watch what you eat and drink and it's best not to talk about your diet. If your hostess thinks you don't like her cooking, explain you feel better when you consume fewer calories.

24. Drinking cold water with meals is a bad habit.
   True.

Cold water reduces the body temperature and makes it more difficult for food to be burned up properly; it imposes a burden on your digestive system.

25. Acid fruits cause "acid stomach" and aid digestion.
   True—depending upon the combination of food.

Acid fruits are considered by some to cause, and by others to cure, "acid stomach." The stomach secretes hydrochloric acid, which is a much stronger acid than citric. An "acid stomach" is essential for good digestion.

26. Prunes and figs are "sure cure" for constipation.
   False—but they can help.

Constipation is normally best combated by eating "high residue" fruits and vegetables. Dried fruits, lettuce, leafy vegetables are especially useful in combating and preventing constipation, but no one food is indispensable or represents a "sure cure." Prunes and figs should be included in the diet because they taste good and provide other benefits.

27. Some people are "naturally fat."
   False.

There are fat families just as there are lean ones. If both parents are overweight, about 70 percent of the children will be obese. If one parent only is fat, then only 10 percent of the children will be obese. In 60 to 80 percent of all cases a family tendency to family history of that condition. In most cases a family tendency to fat has no more mysterious origins than a liking for "setting a good table"; good digestion, or an easy-going and inactive temperment, combined with food habits such as a preference for sweets and fatty foods: and/or a faulty appestat so that a person does not feel satisfied until the stomach is unduly full.

28. No one should attempt to lose weight after 70.

   False.

   Unless a person is suffering from some rare disease where dieting of any kind is to be avoided, no obese person is too old to benefit from weight reduction. In fact, bringing weight down to an "ideal" level is the best way to put "more life into your years"; but drastic, quick-weight-loss, one-dimensional diets *must* be avoided. A diet containing all six "key elements" is imperative.

29. Toasting bread reduces the calories.

   False.

   Toasting bread only reduces the water content. The calorie count remains the same.

30. Starch-reduced spaghetti is not fattening.

   False—if you eat too much of it.

   For practical purposes, starch-reduced spaghetti and macaroni have as many calories as "regular" spaghetti and macaroni.

31. Sour cream contains less calories than sweet cream.

   False.

   Sour cream and sweet cream contain the same number of calories.

32. Margarine has a lower calorie count than butter.

   False.

   The calorie count is the same.

33. Dieters should avoid vitamins before meals.

   True—for some.

   To avoid the appetite-stimulating effects of some vitamins, notably the B-complex vitamins, dieters should take them after meals, washed down with hot water.

34. The practice of meditation twice daily will help people

reduce and keep weight off.

True—according to research and to numerous informal reports and "case histories" of Harbor Island Spa visitors.

Different meditation techniques can be employed with success. There is the meditation technique where a single word—any word—is said over and over, together with gentle effort to eliminate thoughts from the mind. This technique has been shown in various medical studies to produce a variety of benefits, including lowered metabolism; lowered blood pressure; lowered oxygen consumption, reduced airway resistance (a fact of particular importance to those with respiratory problems, including asthma); decreased rate of respiration to as low as four breaths per minute; increased skin resistance (a measure of the electrical properties of the skin thought to be affected by the amount of moisture on the skin surface); and a measurably increased degree of relaxation—deeper than occurs in sleep or under hypnosis.

Chapter 7

Most Commonly Asked Questions

THE more you know about how your body works and the relationship between food, vitamins, minerals, and your emotions to your good health, happiness, and good looks, the more rapidly you'll train that appestat in your brain to demand less food—just enough to match your energy output.

At Harbor Island Spa people may pay hundreds and, in many cases, thousands of dollars to learn the "secrets" of losing fat and keeping it off, the "secrets" of nutrition, and how to enjoy exercise and gain the benefits thereof.

Besides our program of sports and dancing and dance and exercise classes, at Harbor Island Spa we have lectures once or twice a week to which all guests are invited and at which they are encouraged to speak out and ask questions. Here are some of the most frequently asked questions:

Question: "How soon can I expect to reach my ideal weight?"

Answer: There's no one answer to that. It depends upon your starting point, how much you want to lose, your bones, your emotional attitude, your activity pattern, you emotions, and how determined you are to lose.

Question: "I eat faster and longer than others, but I never feel full even when I stop eating out of embarrassment. Why should that be?"

Answer: Because your appestat, over the years, has been trained to demand more food than your activity pattern requires. Even if your appestat did register at the satiety point, the message doesn't get through to your brain fast enough to stop you from lifting fork or spoon to your mouth. While some messages are instantaneous, the appestat requires about 20 minutes to reflect the

71

fullness of the stomach. You can consume a lot of calories in 20 minutes—especially when you are eating fast. Eating fast is the first hazard the dieter must overcome.

Question: "How am I supposed to learn to eat slowly? I'm a nervous person. I do everything fast."

Answer: Practice one trick. Eat one mouthful at a time. Put your fork or spoon on your plate after each mouthful. Don't pick it up again until you have chewed your food well and emptied your mouth.

Question: "Do you allow us to eat bread?"

Answer: We encourage our dieters to substitute artichoke (Jerusalem artichoke) breadsticks available internationally in health food stores. (See Resource List on page). We use such bread sticks crumbled for recipes that call for "breading."

Question: "What assurance do I have that I'll be able to keep the fat off when I leave Harbor Island Spa?"

Answer: Your *will* to keep fat off is your guarantee. We will teach you tricks to slow down your food consumption, give you menus and low-calorie recipes, name low-calorie snacks, but, in the ultimate, it will depend upon your *desire* to keep the fat off.

Question: "Aren't some people happier when they are fat?"

Answer: No. Not if they are really fat—if, when they pinch the flesh along their rib cage, they gather in an inch and one-half or more of fat. How much a person should weigh for optimum health (and therefore happiness) will depend largely upon the bone structure. A heavy-framed, heavy-boned man with well-developed muscles can be in perfect health at 200 pounds whereas a small-boned man of the same height could be at his best weight at 150.

Question: "Do you recommend vitamins or do vitamins play a role in obesity correction?"

Answer: We recommend that every dieter take vitamins to help create a normal, healthy internal environment. Every fat person needs extra help to achieve the promptest possible stabilization of his appestat.

Chapter 8

Vitamins, Minerals, and Enzymes

BECAUSE the majority of fat people are actually suffering from malnutrition, we recommend a minimum number of minerals and vitamin supplements daily—at the very least a high-quality combination vitamin containing the basics. But because it is impossible for any company to create a supplement that satisfies the needs of everyone, we recommend that the person interested in achieving optimum health finds out just what function vitamins, minerals, and enzymes perform.

Since some vitamins stimulate the appetite, we recommend that dieters take food supplements after meals. Interestingly, it has been established that an animal with a low level of vitamin B_1 will have a deranged appestat, and the animal will cease to eat. Once the animal is supplied with B_1, its appetite is restored. That's why we suggest it is safer for the dieter to take vitamins after meals. Those with special needs should augment the basics with supplements designed to aid in their particular conditions, whether it be heart problem, acne, respiratory complaints, diabetes, or other specific problem.

Vitamins and minerals cannot be produced by the body and must be obtained from foods or supplements. Working together with protein, vitamins and minerals enable the body to obtain energy from food; to build new tissue; to synthesize needed chemicals; to allow normal functioning of the digestive tract; to promote nervous stability, resistance to bacterial infection, and metabolism of energy elements. Vitamins act as catalysts in the body—speeding a chemical reaction without taking part in it.

Only small amounts of vitamins are required. Water-soluble vitamins are required daily, since, after performing their function, they are voided from the body. Fat-soluble vitamins—A, D, and

73

E—can be stored and used later, but a better practice is to make sure that your intake is on a daily basis. Minerals are required only in minute amounts and can be stored in the body, but it is not unusual for doctors to find people suffering from mineral deficiencies—notably women and notably in relation to iron.

In theory, we should be able to obtain all the vitamins and minerals we need from the food we eat. In actuality, due to poor soil conditions and other factors, we need outside help. The quantity of nutrients found in food varies, depending upon climatic conditions, the food that animals were fed, the kinds of fertilizers used, the way the food was processed, the cooking methods, and, in the case of fruits and vegetables, how long it has been since they were picked and if they were picked ripe or unripened, and other factors. The method of cooking can affect the vitamin/mineral content of meat, fish, and poultry too. In some cases maturity of the product can have an effect. For instance, mature carrots contain more vitamin A than "baby" carrots. Tomatoes grown in the sun contain more vitamin C than those grown in the shade. Tomatoes ripened on the vine in virgin soil contain more vitamin C than those picked green and allowed to ripen after picking.

VITAMINS

Vitamin A

Vitamin A, fat-soluble, is stored in the liver. You can manage without a new supply of vitamin A for weeks, but if your diet is very low in protein, Vitamin A cannot be released from the liver into the bloodstream.

Vitamin A builds and strengthens mucous membranes, particularly those around the eyes. A deficiency of this vitamin can cause "visual purple" (night blindness), which is the eyes' inability to readjust after being struck by bright light.

Vitamin A's functions are not completely known but some nutritionists believe that lack of Vitamin A may cause arthritic conditions. Vitamin A has been used in doses up to 150,000 units a day to treat acne—but for a restricted period, not exceeding four weeks.

One serving of liver can easily supply a minimum quantity of vitamin A for a week. Broccoli, spinach, beef, poultry, cantaloupe, and peaches are good sources of vitamin A.

74

B₁ (Thiamine)

Thiamine—B₁—is essential to maintain good muscle tone, good nerves, and good functioning of the digestive tract, three vital keys to looking well and feeling well while losing weight. Vitamin B, most important in metabolism of carbohydrates, is absorbed from the intestines and carried to the tissues. Small amounts are stored in your liver, kidneys, muscles, and brain but only enough to maintain optimum functioning of the body for a short period, so that a new supply is needed every day.

The tissues use up only what they need. Since this is a water-soluble vitamin, most unused B₁ is excreted in the urine.

Overcooking of foods, and cooking at too high a heat, can cause severe loss of B₁. Pork, however, while one of the richest sources of B₁, must be thoroughly cooked to eliminate any danger from the trichina worm—a parasite that can be found in pork and that affects the muscles.

Lack of B₁ has been implicated in mental depression, irritability, confusion, loss of memory, inability to concentrate, sensitivity to noise, and malfunction of the cells in the hypothalamus of the brain.

B₁ is found in carrots, asparagus, organ meats, whole wheat and other cereals.

B₂ (Riboflavin)

Vitamin B₂ is used for oxidation processes in various body tissues. It is active in keeping the color and structure tissue of your lips and helps maintain healthy eyes. A lack of B₂ can cause eyes to itch and burn, lips to become pale and to split at the corners of the mouth. There is evidence too that an inadequate supply of B₂ can cause mental depression.

Milk contains generous amounts of B₂, but riboflavin is destroyed quickly by light. If milk is left in glass bottles and exposed to sunlight, much of the riboflavin is lost.

Organ meats, green leafy vegetables, eggs, and fortified cereals are also good sources of B₂, as are yeast and rice bran.

B₃ (Niacin)

Vitamin B_3 aids in the metabolism of carbohydrates and helps living cells generate energy, and so is very important in weight control. Various studies over the last 20 years demonstrate that niacin in mega doses is therapeutic in reducing cholesterol. A deficiency leads to pellagra, a disease marked by inflamed mucous membranes, gastrointestinal disorders, and symptoms of the central nervous system.

Good sources are chicken, veal, tuna, salmon, yeast, and rice bran.

B₆ (Pyridoxine)

B_6, or pyridoxine, consists also of two other forms of the vitamin, pyridoxal and pyridoxamine. This vitamin aids in the breakdown of amino acids and fatty acids in the body, necessary for protein synthesis. Certain doctors have found B_6 extremely helpful in reducing arthritic problems.

B_6 is found in veal, lamb, and a variety of vegetables.

B₁₂ (Cobalamin)

B_{12} is a red crystalline substance that contains phosphorus and cobalt, essential for normal formation of erythrocytes (red blood cells).

Liver, kidney, milk and milk products, and yeast carry different amounts of this vitamin.

Vitamin C (Ascorbic Acid)

Vitamin C is used in the body to cement the body cells together, strengthening the walls of the blood vessels. It forms and maintains capillary walls to prevent pinpoint hemorrhages in the skin that show on the surface as "black and blue" spots. Vitamin C is highly soluble in water, a very good reason to use the smallest amount of water possible when cooking leafy green vegetables and a particularly good reason for eating leafy green vegetables raw as much as possible (and for using the water in which such vegetables are cooked for soups and other purposes).

Vitamin C requirements differ among individuals, some requiring many times what others might need. Some nutritionists recommend ingestion of large amounts of vitamin C for anyone past middle age to reduce various manifestations of aging, including stiffening of the joints.

Research has shown that ascorbic acid, when administered to rats, rabbits, and guinea pigs in large doses has altered blood composition so as to decrease atherosclerosis. Probably the most publicized purported benefit of large amounts of vitamin C is the prevention or cure of the common cold. A less-publicized but vital benefit for those interested in living long and healthily is that ascorbic acid has strong antioxidant properties, and a variety of studies have implicated vitamin C in the causes and control of mental disease. One study showed that, on the average, schizophrenics use ascorbic acid at a rate of 10 times that of normal people. While studies on the relationship of vitamin C to mental disease are inconclusive, there are strong indication that an ample supply is one way to help insure that the brain will function well. Scurvy is a disease representative of a severe vitamin C deficiency.

Citrus fruits, tomatoes, broccoli, and raw leafy vegetables are high in vitamin C.

Vitamin D

Vitamin D, fat soluble, aids in absorption and metabolism of calcium and phosphorus to produce healthy bones. A deficiency causes the bones to become pliable and leads to deformities such as bowlegs and knock-knees.

Good sources for vitamin D, which, like vitamin A, is stored in the liver, include fish oils, milk, cream, butter, and eggs.

Vitamin E (Tocopherol)

Vitamin E was found by feeding fresh dry leaves, or dried alfalfa, to sterile animals with resulting restoration of reproductivity in the female. The known factor that prevented and cured sterility was first known as Substance X and later was named vitamin E.

This is the only fat-soluble vitamin not stored in the liver, but it protects vitamins A and D from oxidation both in the digestive tract and in the body cells. In the human being it has been used in the prevention and treatment of miscarriages, for male and female infertility, and for menopausal and menstrual disorders. It restores male potency.

Used in combination with vitamin C, it is said to enchance vitamin C's effectiveness in the prevention and cure of the common cold: and its most famous use has been in connection with cardiovascular problems. It is effective in heart disease because it dilates the blood vessels. It aids circulation and has been recommended as insurance against premature aging. It is used by certain nutritionally minded doctors in the treatment of asthma, emphysema, hypoglycemia, leg ulcers, phlebitis, varicose veins, and a variety of other problems. Its use on the skin prevents and heals scar tissue formation from burns, sores, and surgery.

Wheat germ is a pure form of vitamin E. It is also found in liver, egg yolk, and corn oil.

Vitamin F

While vitamin F (essential fatty acids) has been found to be essential to good health, no minimum daily requirement, or optimum level, has been established as yet. Medical research indicates that vitamin F is important in the prevention of heart disease by lowering blood cholesterol. It is deemed essential for normal glandular activity, particularly of the adrenal glands, and it is needed for many metabolic processes as well as for healthy skin and mucous membranes.

Sources include vegetable oils, such as soybean, corn, safflower, and sunflower.

Vitamin P (Bioflavonoids)

Bioflavonoids strengthen capillary walls and prevent or correct capillary fragility and prevent capillary hemorrhaging. It acts as an anticoagulant. It has been found to be beneficial in hypertension, infections, hemorrhoids, respiratory infections, bleeding gums, eczema, psoriasis, cirrhosis of the liver, coronary thrombosis, and arteriosclerosis.

Appearance of purplish or blue spots on the skin is a symptom of a deficiency.

Sources include fresh fruits and vegetables, green peppers, grapes, apricots, citrus fruits, currants, cherries, and prunes. Bioflavonoids are largely destroyed by cooking.

MINERALS

A healthy body exists in a state of equal mineral balance, with the intake balancing the excretion. The body needs only "trace" minerals for good health; they are essential, yet great care should be taken before supplementing the diet with any isolated minerals, particularly the "trace minerals," since the body's chemistry can be upset by an undue intake of any one of several minerals.

Among the minerals that are essential to vital functions of the body are:

Calcium (Ca)

Calcium is needed to build bones and teeth and for normal growth; it is important for heart action, muscle activity, and all the healing processes. It is needed for normal clotting of the blood and for many enzyme functions.

Deficiency symptoms include tooth decay, rickets, nervousness, mental depression, muscle cramps and spasm, insomnia, irritability, heart palpitation, retarded growth, and porous and fragile bones.

Calcium sources include milk and cheese; most raw vegetables, particularly dark-green leafy vegetables such as lettuce, watercress, dandelion greens, endive, kale, cabbage, broccoli, and Brussels sprouts. Other sources include oats, Navy beans, sunflower seeds, walnuts, almonds, and sesame seeds. Calcium lactate and bone meal are natural supplements.

Phosphorus (P)

Phosphorus works together with calcium. They must be in proper ratio to be effective. Phosphorus is important in carbohydrate metabolism and in maintaining a proper acid-alkaline balance in blood and tissues. It is needed for healthy nerves, efficient mental activity, building bones and maintaining healthy teeth. Sources include nuts, seeds, whole grains, dairy products, egg yolks, corn, dried fruits, and fish.

Magnesium (Mg)

Magnesium helps in the utilization of vitamins B and E, fats, calcium and other minerals, and in efficient synthesis of protein. An important catalyst in many enzyme actions, magnesium prevents build-up of blood cholesterol. It is a natural tranquilizer.

Sources include cooked green leafy vegetables, especially beet tops: chard, celery, endive, and kale. It is also found in figs, apples, lemons, almonds, sunflower seeds, sesame seeds, brown rice, and peaches.

Chlorine (Cl)

Chlorine is essential for the production of hydrochloric acid in the stomach, which is required for both protein digestion and assimilation of minerals. Chlorine aids the detoxifying activity of the liver and is involved in maintenance of proper electrolyte and fluid balance in the system.

Sources include avocado, tomatoes, cabbage, kale, endive, turnip, celery, cucumber, asparagus, salt-water fish, pineapple, watercress, and kelp.

Copper (Cu)

Copper is essential for the absorption of iron. Copper aids in development of brain, bones, nerves, and connective tissues, and is involved in protein metabolism, healing processes, and in hair color-retention. Deficiency may cause anemia, hair loss, digestive disturbances, heart damage, and impaired respiration.

Good sources are almonds, beans, peas, green leafy vegetables, liver, raisins, and prunes.

Iron (Fe)

Iron is essential for the formation of the hemoglobin that carries oxygen from the lungs to every cell of the body. Iron increases resistance to stress and disease and builds up the quality of the blood. Iron deficiency may result in anemia, shortness of breath, headaches, diminished sexual drive, pale complexion, and a general feeling of being "run down."

Good sources of iron are prunes, raisins, apricots, peaches, bananas, brewer's yeast, whole-grain cereals, spinach, beets, turnip greens, walnuts, sesame seeds, dry beans, lentils, kelp, liver, egg yolks.

Iodine (I)

Iodine is essential for the formation of thyroxin, the thyroid hormone that regulates much of physical and mental activity. Iodine regulates the rate of metabolism, energy production, and body weight and so is a mineral of particular interest to the obese.

A deficiency may cause goiter, anemia, fatigue, lethargy, diminished sexual interest, low blood pressure, and rough and wrinkled skin. A serious deficiency can result in high blood cholesterol and heart disease.

Natural sources of iodine include Swiss chard, turnip greens, garlic, watercress, artichokes, pineapple, pears, citrus fruits, egg yolks, seafood, fish liver oils, kelp, dulse, and other seaweed.

Manganese (Mn)

Manganese is an important component of several enzymes that are involved in the metabolism of carbohydrates, fats, and proteins. Combined with choline, manganese aids fat digestion and utilization. It helps to nourish the brain and nerves and aids in proper coordination between brain, nerves, and muscles. Deficiencies can produce digestive disturbances, sterility, poor equilibrium, and abnormal bone development. Manganese deficiencies have been implicated by certain researchers in asthma and myasthenia gravis.

Good sources are spinach, beets, Brussels sprouts, green leafy vegetables, apricots, blueberries, grapefruit, oranges, peas, raw egg yolk, wheat germ, kelp, nuts, and whole grains.

Fluorine (F)

Fluorine protects against infections and is essential for bone and tooth building. It has been called an internal antiseptic.

Sources include sunflower seeds, milk, cheese, carrots, garlic, green vegetables, beet tops, and steel-cut oats.

Molybdenum (Mo)

Molybdenum is an integral part of selected enzymes, particularly those involved with oxidation processes and carbohydrate metabolism.

Sources include naturally hard water, brown rice, millet, buckwheat, brewer's yeast, and legumes.

Potassium (K)

Potassium is an alkalizing agent important in keeping proper acid-alkaline balance in blood and tissues. Potassium is important for proper heart function; it promotes the secretion of hormones, stimulates endocrine hormone production, is involved in proper functioning of the nervous system, and aids the kidneys in detoxifying the blood. A severe depletion can cause muscle weakness and even heart failure.

Natural sources include all vegetables, but particularly leafy green vegetables: bananas, avocados, persimmons, oranges, milk, yogurt, nuts, whole grains, white and sweet potatoes, mushrooms; also poultry, meat, and fish.

Sodium (Na)

Sodium, together with potassium and chlorine, helps maintain proper electrolyte balance. The three minerals, which function by changing into electrically charged ions that transport nerve impulses, control and maintain osmotic pressure that is responsible for transportation of nutrients from the intestines into the blood. Sodium plays a part in many glandular secretions. It is essential for hydrochloric acid production in the stomach.

Sulfur (S)

Sulfur is involved in oxidation reduction processes and is vital for healthy skin, hair, and nails. Symptoms of deficiency include skin disorders like eczema and blemishes. Brittle nails are another symptom.

Natural sources include celery, radishes, turnips, onions, string beans, watercress, soybeans, kale, horseradish, fish, and meat.

Lithium (Li)

Lithium is involved in sodium metabolism and its transportation in nerves and muscles. It is associated with function of the autonomic or involuntary nervous system.

Kelp and sea water are natural sources.

Selenium (Se)

Selenium is an antioxidant. Closely related to utilization of vitamin E, it can help in regeneration of the liver and it has been suggested that it may slow the aging processes by inhibiting formation of free radicals. Sources include garlic, mushrooms, seafoods, milk, eggs, most vegetables, cereals, brewer's yeast, and kelp.

The minimum daily requirement has not been established but it has been found to be toxic in overdoses.

Cobalt (Co)

Cobalt is necessary for the synthesis of vitamin B_{12}. Cobalt aids in hemoglobin formation. A deficiency can lead to pernicious anemia.

Liver and all green leafy vegetables are natural sources.

Chromium (Cr)

Chromium is an integral part of many enzymes and hormones and is a cofactor with insulin to move glucose from the blood into the cells. It is essential for proper utilization of sugar, it is important in cholesterol metabolism, and it is involved in the synthesis of heart protein.

Chromium is present normally in natural waters, particularly in highly mineralized waters. It is found in whole-grain bread, liver, mushrooms, and raw sugar.

Silicon (Si)

Silicon is beneficial in all healing processes and is essential for building bones and for normal growth of hair, nails, and teeth. Silicon protects against many diseases, including irritations in mucous membranes, skin diseases, and tuberculosis.

Natural sources include apples, strawberries, grapes, onions, beets, almonds, peanuts, sunflower seeds, and parsnips.

Zinc (Zn)

Zinc is essential for the synthesis of body protein and is involved in many enzyme and hormone activities. Required in the construction of insulin, it is involved in carbohydrate, energy, and vitamin A metabolism, and it affects respiration. It is essential for normal growth and development of sex organs and normal function of the prostate gland.

Zinc speeds healing after burns and wounds and it is essential for bone formation. Deficiency symptoms include white spots on finger and toe nails and reduced senses of smell and taste.

Good sources of zinc are onions, oysters, nuts, herring, green leafy vegetables, milk, eggs, wheat germ, wheat bran, sunflower seeds, and pumpkin seeds.

NUTRITIONAL SUPPLEMENTS

Since it is difficult to select supplements that fill all needs, we recommend at Harbor Island Spa use of a vitamin/mineral supplement containing varying amounts of the following:

Vitamins A, D, C, Thiamine, Riboflavin, Pyridoxine, Niacin, Pantothenic Acid, vitamin B_{12}, vitamin E, and the following minerals: calcium, phosphorus, magnesium, cobalt, copper, iodine, iron, manganese, molybdenum, and zinc.

We also recommend taking individual capsules—or tablets—of vitamin A, vitamin C, and vitamin E, and suggest consideration to augmenting the natural diet with a B-complex capsule and, if any arthritic condition is present, an extra B_6 tablet.

ENZYMES

Enzymes are produced by living cells. Essential to life, they act as catalysts in promoting a variety of processes, including oxidation. Cooking fruits and vegetables destroys enzymes—a basic reason to be sure that you eat some raw fruits and vegetables daily.

BASIC NUTRITIONAL REQUIREMENTS

You have already learned that the human body requires six basic nutrients:
1. Carbohydrates
2. Fats
3. Protein
4. Vitamins
5. Minerals
6. Water

Carbohydrates include such popular foods as sugar, cereals, flour, bread, cake, cookies, rice, potatoes, spaghetti, macaroni. Most fruits and vegetables contain some carbohydrate. Carbohydrates and fats provide energy and if your carbohydrate-fat intake is insufficient to fulfill your energy requirements, protein will be utilized for energy.

You need a daily supply of carbohydrates because this nutrient cannot be stored for any length of time—12 to 24 hours at the most. One missed meal can use up all the carbohydrates you have in storage. Those not used for energy or temporary storage turn into body fat. Regulate your carbohydrate-fat intake by your total caloric allowance, but do not choose foods for their carbohydrate content alone. Foods rich in protein, vitamins, and minerals also furnish carbohydrates.

Fats not used for energy can be stored for later use, but consistent intake of fat over energy requirements rapidly produces body fat. However, keep in mind that fats provide essential fatty acids necessary for the maintenance of body functions, so be sure to include some fat in your diet daily—at the very least a teaspoonful on a salad.

You need carbohydrates and fat daily to ensure that protein is not used to supply your energy needs. Protein has a more important role to play in your body. Protein provides enzymes to aid digestion and aids your body in resisting disease; it makes up about four-fifths of muscle tissue and provides materials to build, maintain, and repair body cells. Protein is an essential part of every cell, furnishing the cells with nitrogen. Protein is the only nutrient that provides nitrogen, and without nitrogen the cells of the body will die. Cell-building starts with nitrogen. Since thousands of cells are dying in your body right at this instant, the importance of having enough protein in the diet becomes clear. As a nation, we are known as protein-eaters, yet statistics show that approximately one-fourth of the U.S. population does not have enough protein in its diet.

Protein is best assimilated if it is acquired in three daily portions—a good reason the one-meal-a-day fad diet is quite harmful. Protein provides the body with amino acids, essential to the cell-building function. Scientists have determined that there are 22 amino acids, 14 of which can be manufactured within the body if there is a sufficient supply of nitrogen. The other eight amino acids have been labeled "essential" because studies show that if any one of these eight is absent from the diet a negative nitrogen balance is produced in the body and cell building does not take place.

Research by Dr. William C. Rose of the University of Illinois showed that all eight of the essential amino acids have to be present in the body *simultaneously* for there to be cell building. The cell-building process takes place immediately after each meal, Dr. Rose determined, and there is, disturbingly, no carry-over of supplies of amino acids from one meal to the next. This is a basic and sound reason why three meals a day should be considered essential and minimal and why so many people—probably a majority of them if truth were known—function best when they ingest three modest-sized meals and three other smaller meals, or nutritious snacks between meals (and that does not mean "coffee and Danish"!).

Astonishingly, only six foods provide all eight of the essential amino acids: meat, fish, eggs, cheese, milk, and soybeans. These six are called "complete proteins." And you need only one of the complete proteins to be certain that the cell-building process will take place—an excellent reason to have a complete protein at breakfast, and why "Coffee and Cigarette" is disastrous. It is a very good reason why you should have a complete protein at lunch. If you are practicing "eating like a pauper" at supper or dinner, be sure you include at least a glass of milk or put soybeans in your salad.

Your body can acquire complete protein another way: when you successfully combine two complementary "incomplete proteins." Two or more incomplete proteins can cause the cell-building function to operate providing the combination provides all eight of the essential amino acids. But, as of now, there is no source that will tell you how to combine incomplete proteins to provide the eight essentials. Incomplete protein is utilized in the cell-building process, of course, but only if there is adequate nitrogen present and that comes only when the eight essential amino acids are present simultaneously.

Incomplete proteins include bread and gelatin. There are two grams of incomplete protein in an average slice of white bread or 3 percent of the body's daily protein requirement. Gelatin provides about four grams in an average serving. By itself, gelatin will not help build cells in your body. Combined with fish in a jellied salad or with milk or eggs in a dessert, gelatin extends the cell-building process set in motion by the fish, milk, or eggs.

The Recommended Daily Allowance of protein set by the National Academy of Sciences is

Children ....1–10 years..........25–40 grams
Boys ....10–18 years ....45–60 grams
Girls.................10–18 years ....50–55 grams
Adult men...........18 and over.........60–65 grams
Adult women ....18 and over ....55 grams

When you select one complete protein at each meal you can be sure you are getting your daily requirement. Since you must be concerned with total calorie intake, guide your protein selection according to the calories. Then you'll be sure you're building your cells while trimming off the fat.

You aren't going to collapse if you go a meal or a day without ingesting a complete protein, but if you were to do it day after day you are in for trouble. Your cells will not be replaced as they should be. Your body will become less resistant to disease and infection.

From conception until death, the body and the brain require a frequent and regular supply of complete protein. In the following table, from Agriculture Handbook No. 456 of the Agricultural

Research Service, U.S. Department of Agriculture, you will see a listing of the protein values of complete and incomplete proteins, together with the weight in grams and the caloric, fat, and carbohydrate values, since all three are essential for the person on a diet. The table below is incomplete but provides a sampling of commonly eaten foods. C indicates complete protein; I, incomplete protein.

COMPLETE AND INCOMPLETE PROTEINS

Food	Grams	Measure	Calories	Protein (grams)	Fat (grams)	Carbo-hydrate (grams)
Peanuts	144	1 cup	838	37.7 I	70.1	29.7
Cottage Cheese (dry curd)	200	1 cup	172	34 C	.6	5.4
Turkey (white meat)	85	3 oz.	162	26.8C	5.2	0
Turkey (dark meat)	85	3 oz.	173	25.5 C	7.1	0
Tuna (canned/water)	184	6.25 oz.	234	51.5 C	1.5	0
Tuna (canned/oil)	184	6.25 oz.	530	44.5 C	37.7	0
Rump roast beef	85	3 oz.	177	24.7 C	7.9	0
Beef steak	85	3 oz.	212	24.6 C	11.8	0
Chipped beef	71	2.5 oz.	144	24.4 C	4.5	0
Almonds	130	1 cup	777	24.2 I	70.6	0
Cheese, Swiss	85	3 oz.	315	23.4 C	23.7	1.5
Salmon (canned)	220	6.25 oz.	447	47.7 C	26.8	0
Veal roast	85	3 oz.	229	23.1 C	14.4	0
Liver, beef	85	3 oz.	195	22.4 C	9.0	4.5
Swordfish	85	3 oz.	138	22.2 C	7.4	1.6
Bluefish (broiled, butter)	85	3 oz.	135	22.2 C	4.5	0
Lamb (leg)	85	3 oz.	237	21.5 C	16.1	0
Lamb chops, loin	95	3.4oz.	341	20.9C	27.9	0

Food	Grams	Measure	Calories	Protein (grams)	Fat (grams)	Carbo-hydrate (grams)
Roast pork	85	3 oz.	308	20.8 C	24.2	0
Corned beef, canned	80	2 slices	172	20.2 C	9.6	0
Soybeans	180	1 cup	234	19.8C	10.3	19.4
Roast ham	85	3 oz.	318	19.6 C	26.0	0
Spaghetti, with cheese,meatballs, tomato sauce	248	1 cup	332	18.6 C	11.7	38.7
Lamb shoulder	85	3 oz.	287	18.4 C	23.1	0
walnuts (pieces)	120	1 cup	781	17.8 I	76.8	19.0
Sardines (canned/oil)	85	3 oz.	264	17.4 C	20.7	.6
Rib roast	85	3 oz.	374	16.9 C	33.5	0
Macaroni & cheese	200	1 cup	430	16.8 C	22.2	40.2
Roast chicken	50	2 pieces	83	15.8 C	1.7	0
Beans, kidney	185	1 cup	218	14.4 I	.9	39.6
Beans, lima	170	1 cup	189	12.9 I	.9	89.8
Broccoli, boiled	280	1 lge. stalk	73	8.7 I	.8	12.6
Milk, whole	244	1 cup	159	8.5 C	8.5	12.0
Milk, skim	245	1 cup	88	8.8 C	.2	12.5
Milk, canned, unsweetened evaporated	252	1 cup	345	17.6 C	19.2	24.4
Milk, dry nonfat	120	1 cup	436	43.1 C	1.0	62.8
Yogurt, partly skim milk	245	1 cup	123	8.3 C	4.2	12.7
Goat's milk	244	1 cup	163	7.8 C	9.8	11.2
Yogurt, whole milk	245	1 cup	152	7.4 C	8.3	12.0
Oysters (raw)	85	3 oz.	57	7.2 C	1.5	3.0
Cheese, cream	85	3 oz.	318	6.8 C	32.0	1.8
Gelatin, dry	27	1 envelope	23.75	6.07 I	Trace	--
Brussels sprouts	155	1 cup	56	6.5 I	.6	9.9
Cheese, American, processed	27	1 slice	100	6.3 C	8.1	.5
Spinach, boiled	180	1 cup	41	5.4 I	.5	6.5
Oatmeal	240	1 cup	132	4.8 I	2.4	23.3

Food	Grams	Measure	Calories	Protein (grams)	Fat (grams)	Carbo-hydrate (grams)
Artichokes	380	1 bud	60	4.3 I	.8	15.0
Asparagus, cooked, whole	180	1 cup	36	4.0 I	.4	6.5
Squash, winter, baked	205	1 cup	139	3.7 I	.2	35.9
Sweet potato, boiled in skin	180	1 potato	172	2.6 I	.6	39.8
Sweet Potato baked in skin	146	1 potato	161	2.4 I	.6	37.0
Avocado	125	½	188	2.4 I	18.5	7.1
Bread, whole wheat	25	1 slice	61	2.6 I	.8	11.9
Bread, rye	25	1 slice	61	2.3 I	.3	13.0
Bread, white enriched	25	1 slice	63	2.1 I	.9	11.5
Spinach, raw	55	1 cup	14	1.8 I	.2	2.4

Chapter 9

Calorie Counting and Special Diets

SOME people will take the time and make the effort to weigh their food before they cook it or otherwise prepare it. Others simply prefer to guess. While we recommend weighing your food, we also know that you will very soon be able to estimate quite accurately how large a piece of fish is represented by three ounces and what constitutes one gram.

Since no one expects you to sit down and calculate your diet to meet the standards to which nutritionists must conform, you should keep in mind a few simple guidelines:

1 gram of carbohydrates yields 4 calories
1 gram of protein yields 4 calories
1 gram of fat yields 9 calories
30 grams equal 1 ounce.

An 8-ounce glass of whole milk represents 158.5 calories, divided in this wise:

Carbohydrate	12 grams × 4 =	48
Protein	8.5 grams × 4 =	34
Fat	8.5 grams × 9 =	76.5
Total Calories		158.5

In the table in Chapter 8, the calories are listed as 159, but for convenience in adding in planning the day's caloric intake, we normally list the caloric value of an 8-ounce glass of milk at 160.

To achieve the Minimum Daily Requirement of 60 grams of protein (two ounces) for adult men and 55 grams of protein for adult women, you allocate, for men 240 calories; for women, 220 calories. If you want to restrict your fat intake to approximately one-third your daily caloric allowance, and assuming you are a male on a maintenance diet of 1600 calories daily, you should restrict your ingestion of fat to about 60 grams per day.

There are three kinds of fat: saturated, polyunsaturated, and monosaturated. Monosaturated is fat that is neutral and neither raises nor lowers blood cholesterol levels. Olive oil, peanuts, peanut oil, and peanut butter are monsaturated.

Foods high in saturated fats include beef, veal, lamb, pork, sausages, organ meats, egg yolks, whole milk, whole milk cheese (American, Swiss, and other hard cheeses), cream and cream cheese, ice cream, butter, some margarines, solid shortenings, chocolate, coconut, coconut oil, and foods prepared with any of these products, including most cakes, cookies, and gravies.

Foods high in polyunsaturated fat include fish, mayonnaise, liquid oils of vegetable origin and margarines containing substantial amounts of liquid vegetable oils. Turkey and chicken contain both saturated and unsaturated fat in almost equal proportions. California walnuts, per 100 grams, contained 46.5 grams of polyunsaturated and 17.5 grams of saturated fat. When polyunsaturated fats are substituted for part of the saturated fats in the diet, the blood cholesterol is lowered. As yet there is no proof that a diet low in unsaturated fat will prevent a heart attack, but many researchers believe it may reduce the risk.

Even lean meat contains saturated fat. To reduce intake of saturated fat, use a rack to drain off the fat when broiling, roasting, or baking. If the recipe calls for basting, instead of drippings use bouillon, tomato juice, or wine. Cook stews, boiled meat, soup stock, and other dishes in which fat cooks into the liquid a day ahead of serving, refrigerate overnight and skim hardened fat from the top before reheating. Broil lamb chops, steak, pork chops, and hamburger rather than pan-frying such meats.

To further restrict your saturated fat intake, choose lean cuts of meat, trim visible fat, and limit your intake of beef, lamb, pork, and ham to no more than five moderate portions per week, choosing, instead, fish, poultry, and veal. Severely temper your use of "variety" meats such as salami, sausages, and so forth.

Watching your cholesterol levels and controlling your weight are basic contributions you can make to your good health but they do not substitute for regular checkups by your physician. If you are seriously overweight and have any question at all about your health, we urge you to see your physician before you begin any radical change in your life style. That way you can take into consideration any special needs or problems you may have. We have resident physicians (and nurses) at Harbor Island Spa and many of our guests have a medical checkup at the start of their stay with us.

When a nutritional imbalance has persisted for a considerable time, the results are not usually quickly reversed. Indeed, the condition may be so severe that the victim may find it necessary to control his diet carefully for the rest of his life. But that does not mean that he does not have plenty of good, tasty, delicious food to choose from—and to serve to friends and relatives without any of them ever knowing they are being treated to a "special diet."

Even in a "salt free" diet, it is easy to serve foods without anyone realizing that salt has been excluded from every dish. There are other ways besides salt to ensure taste sparkle for even the blandest foods. And the more restrictions there are on salt, the more the distinctive flavors of the foods will be recognized and appreciated.

One of the worst habits of Americans, and one that will raise the hackles of almost any good cook, is salting food before tasting it. That habit does two things: destroys the cook's special effort to use just the right amount of salt (if any) for a particular dish, and it blunts the taste buds so that individual flavors are lost in a cover of salt. The habit of oversalting can lead eventually to a condition where it may be necessary, for health's sake, to eliminate salt from the diet altogether.

SODIUM (SALT)-RESTRICTED DIETS

Often guests at Harbor Island Spa are on sodium (salt)-restricted diets prescribed by their physicians. An essential element of the body, sodium is maintained by osmotic pressure—pressure between two solution of different strengths, which, when a person is healthy, produces the proper balance between the volume of intracellular (inside the cells) and extracellular (outside the cells) fluids.

A person in normal health is able to excrete the sodium not needed by the body through the skin, bowels, and kidneys—mostly the kidneys. In some cases too much sodium is retained and edema—accumulation of extracellular fluids—results. Sodium-restricted diets are used to prevent, control, and eliminate edema. Many times, persons with high blood pressure are put on a salt-restricted diet. In such cases, use of table salt, our most common dietary source of sodium, must be restricted.

Organ meats, shellfish, spinach, kale, sauerkraut, and celery contain large amounts of sodium and so should be omitted from a sodium-restricted diet. Chicken, fresh fish, veal, fresh vegetables (other than those mentioned above), fruits, and unprocessed cereals are recommended. Delicious and healthy substitutes for salt, to enhance the flavor of foods, include herbs, spices, and lemon juice. (See Harbor Island Cookbook.)

FAT-FREE DIET

For those suffering from arteriosclerosis (atherosclerosis), a carefully controlled diet is essential. The condition is characterized by abnormal thickening, hardening, and loss of elasticity of the artery walls, together with the formation of cholesterol plaques (fatty deposits) within the arteries and of triglycerides (a milklike substance from natural body fats) in the blood system.

Cholesterol is a fat-soluble crystalline steroid that occurs as an essential constituent of animal cells and body fluids and is important in physiological processes. Cholesterol is synthesized in the body, particularly in the liver and the adrenal cortex, and is used in the synthesis of Vitamin D and steroid hormones. When cholesterol exceeds what is considered normal, many medical authorities believe that cholesterol-rich foods, such as muscle meats, egg yolks,

93

cream, butter and other saturated fats should be eliminated from the diet.

Some doctors referring patients to the Spa will warn us to watch out for cholesterol level; others put more stress on the triglyceride level. Dr. Abram Hoffer of Saskatchewan, Canada, biochemist, physician, and psychiatrist, is one of the many doctors concerned equally about both and advocates inclusion of 3 grams of niacin (Vitamin B_3) daily to lower cholesterol and triglyceride levels. By lowering the quantity of cholesterol and triglycerides in the body, the blood exerts less pressure on the vessels.

For the person with high blood cholesterol or high triglyceride levels or both, we recommend several small meals instead of three large ones; raw nuts and seeds within the daily caloric restrictions; avoidance of saturated fats in favor of cold-pressed vegetable oils; avoidance of salt, sugar, and white flour; and most particularly we urge anyone with arteriosclerosis to eschew "empty calories" rigorously.

Some doctors and nutritionists urge avoidance of eggs by anyone with arteriosclerosis. Others are not at all sure eggs should be eliminated. Everyone agrees that what is most needed is a low-calorie, highly nutritious diet. Famed biochemist Roger J. Williams points out that cholesterol is an absolute essential for our bodies all through life. Confirming that truly good nutrition will prevent cholesterol deposits from forming, he suggests that the person with arteriosclerosis should consume more lecithin. Lecithin is a powerful emulsifying agent and its presence in the body tends to dissolve cholesterol deposits. One research study showed that cholesterol levels in the blood of participating patients were lowered "substantially" by ingestion of about one ounce of lecithin per day for three months. Lecithin, as cholesterol, is made within the body, but for therapeutic action, supplements are required. Vitamin E, choline, Vitamin B_6, and folic acid are also thought to be in short supply in those suffering from arteriosclerosis.

DIABETIC DIET (SUGAR-FREE)

Diabetes is a condition wherein the body does not efficiently burn the carbohydrates (starches and sugars) in the diet to produce the energy required to keep an active individual going. Usually,

94

under normal conditions, sugars and starches are "split" by intestinal juices into simple substances, such as glucose, the body's own sugar. Part of the glucose goes directly into the bloodstream where is is used as an immediate source of food and energy for every cell in the body. The remaining glucose is converted into another form called glycogen and is stored in the liver.

Insulin is required by the body to burn glucose and so supply energy for the body's needs. Insulin is secreted into the blood by the pancreas, a gland located near the stomach. When insufficient insulin is available, due to poor functioning of the pancreas, glucose is not adequately burned; it builds up in the blood, passes through the kidneys, and appears in the urine. Result: diabetes.

More than 80 of 100 adult diabetics have been overweight before their condition develops. Regardless of the stage of diabetes, which, together with heart disease and cancer, is a primary killer in the United States, the diet should be low in calories and stress vegetables, grains, and fruits. Contrary to popular belief, fruits are beneficial to a diabetic. Fresh fruits contain sugar, called fructose, that does not require insulin to be metabolized and so is well tolerated by diabetics. Grapefruit and banana are strongly recommended, and raw foods of all kinds because raw foods stimulate the pancreas and increase insulin production. For protein, cottage cheese and various forms of soured milks (yogurt, etc.) are recommended; nuts and avocados too, but in small quantities because of their high caloric value. Diabetics have a slowed-down protein and fat metabolism and so have a tendency toward overacidity. The diet should emphasize such alkaline foods as green beans, cucumbers, and Jerusalem artichokes.

While diabetes has been known since Biblical days, it occurs less in poor and underdeveloped countries and often is called a "prosperity" disease because, research indicates, overeating is often a cause. But fasting is not recommended. Most diabetics flourish best on four to six small meals a day. At Harbor Island Spa we use an exchange-system diet that permits an almost endless menu variety. The dietary requirements differ with the individuals according to whether they are taking insulin, and, if so, the type and extent. The carbohydrate content of the diet usually is less than normal while the protein and fat content is somewhat higher, but caution must be exercised because proteins and fats, if eaten to excess, can induce diabetes, or exacerbate it if the condition already exists.

HYPOGLYCEMIC DIET

Hypoglycemia has been called a ''fad'' disease. Many doctors simply refuse to recognize it, even though it has been acknowledged to be one of the most destructive diseases of this country, responsible for such distressing symptoms as excessive fatigue, extreme nervousness, crying jags, and ''passing out'' after the consumption of one or two cocktails. Some physicians blame hypoglycemia for many suicides and even for murderous tendencies.

Hypoglycemia is of two types: functional, sometimes called ''nervous'' hypoglycemia, which is controlled solely through diet, and ''true'' hyperinsulinism (another name for hypoglycemia) that results from an insulin-secreting tumor of the pancreas. Surgery is the only know treatment for the latter condition.

The hypoglycemic obese are benefitted by losing weight, but their diets must be tailored to provide frequent meals to prevent a drop in blood sugar with the subsequent seizures that occur when there is too long a period between meals. The usual impulse of the hypoglycemic suffering a sharp drop in his blood sugar level is to grab something sweet, which provides temporary relief at the cost of aggravating the disease.

Too much insulin produces low blood sugar or hypoglycemia. If the blood sugar falls rapidly, early symptoms are likely to include hunger, weakness, sweating, apprehension, trembling. If the blood sugar falls slowly, early symptoms are more likely to be headache, paresthesia (pins and needles) of the hands and feet, blurring of vision, and drowsiness. Later symptoms, whether of rapid or slow fall of the blood sugar level, include double vision, loss of memory, confusion, and, finally, loss of consciousness, sometimes with convulsions. Some victims have been institutionalized for mental illness, their hypoglycemic state going undetected.

The usual solution is a diet high in fats and/or high in protein and low in carbohydrate. The American Diabetic Association issues a commonly used diet. Certain nutritionists, however, recommend a diet comparatively low in animal protein as well as carbohydrates, but high in milk and milk products, vegetable oils, fruit, vegetables

96

(raw and cooked), and a breakfast including cooked buckwheat or oatmeal served with butter or a tablespoon of vegetable oil. Cooked whole grains release sugars into the blood stream gradually, helping to keep the blood sugar level. Cottage cheese at breakfast is another recommendation. Hypoglycemics should eat five to eight small meals daily. Snacks between meals can be seeds or fruit (provided you eat only one fruit at a time), fruit juice diluted 50 percent with water, vegetable juices, raw vegetables. Nuts could be a regular choice if weight loss were not your goal. Salt should be avoided.

DIET FOR GERIATRICS

We are what we are today largely because of our yesterdays. The older we become, the more yesterdays there are to affect us. However, good nutrition is as necessary in later life as in early years, and one is never too old to start ingesting a more nutritious diet. In later years the ability of the body to handle an excess of food diminishes, and often inadequately chewed foods—the result of poor teeth, badly fitted dentures, or carelessness—place a strain on the digestion. Movement of the alimentary (digestive) system and secretion of digestive juices are slowed down so that the digestive abilities are further enfeebled. The liver, kidneys, other organs and glands are less active or less able to respond to extra work.

Oxidation processes by which foods are utilized in the tissues go on more slowly and sometimes less completely, while the excretion of waste products is more difficult. Because of diminished absorption, a diet higher in protein, vitamins, and minerals is recommended. Fats are often poorly tolerated because they retard gastric evacuation. The blood cholesterol usually becomes elevated as age increases. We recommend obtaining fats from vegetable oils and eating tender vegetables and fruit for fiber.

Chapter 10

Exercise For Health and Beauty and a Healthy Appestat

EXERCISE is the most neglected and misunderstood phase of weight reduction. People don't understand why they should exercise. They forget that their body is like a machine—actually is a machine, the most wonderful and durable in the world. But, like a machine, it "rusts" and becomes creaky if it is not used, not lubricated. Anything that is not used atrophies, which goes for muscles too. If you believe in Darwin's theory, we lost our tails because we stopped using them to swing through the trees. There are those who believe the automobile has set us on the path to losing our feet!

The most important reason for exercise is to make sure your moving parts will keep moving. Exercise is necessary for muscle tone, skin tone, and for a well-functioning digestive system. Metabolizing of fat is improved by exercise. Caloric consumption is related to muscle activity. Your energy expenditure is increased significantly only by a significant increase in the use of muscle. The rate of weight loss is a function of muscle activity but, of course, also must be related to caloric intake. Remember the goal is a healthy appestat where caloric intake automatically matches caloric output (energy output).

Your exercise program must be soundly conceived, related to the current condition of your health. Daily exercise, even as little as 15 minutes a day, is vastly better for you than no exercise Monday through Friday, followed by five hours exercise Saturday and Sunday. That latter route is dangerous. It can be more than dangerous; it can be deadly.

Jeff Paskow, Larry Paskow's younger son, who joined the staff at the Miami Spa in 1976 at age 25 after completing graduate courses in nutrition and hotel management at Cornell University, has a six-days-a-week exercise-fitness program that consists of consumption of fewer calories than at age 18; 15 minutes in the steam room; 20 minutes of exercise; 20 minutes rest (wrapped in a blanket); climaxed by a 5-minute shower starting with hot and alternating with cold, and ending with icy cold.

Even older people will find this system of showering agreeable and beneficial but, in the beginning, anyone can hesitate about the "ice cold" climax. Turn the hot water on for one minute, then cold as you can comfortably stand it for 10 to 20 seconds; then hot, then cold, then hot and cold again.

Such a shower, following exercise, is wonderful for the circulation, but, like exercise, needs to be embarked upon with awareness. In planning your exercise program, a safe rule, if there is no limiting physical condition, is to exercise to the point of first evidence of fatigue. Then stop. After a rest, perhaps 30 minutes or so, wrapped in a blanket if you have become very hot and are sweating, exercise can be resumed, but again must be stopped at the first sign of fatigue.

Only the simplest exercises should be tried initially. As exercise tolerance increases, the amount of activity should be increased and new forms added. Walking is the most natural and best tolerated exercise for the obese. At Harbor Island in Miami, Larry Paskow conducts "walking tours," an idea you and some friends could emulate for pleasure and physical profit.

Exercise improves carbohydrate metabolism and cuts down cholesterol deposits in the blood. Although body *weight* may not change significantly through a daily exercise program, body *shape* most definitely can. In a short time, through a daily exercise program, body fat will diminish and muscle tissue increase, with a dramatic improvement in body composition.

Exercise teaches you how to improve and control the condition of every part of your body. It can be enjoyable for anyone, regardless of age or how much out of condition you may think you are. Almost everyone has some portion of the body that is below par—stiff, tense, or weak. Exercise can overcome these handicaps.

Exercise done in moderation, but done every day, can free you from some tension, help normalize your weight, help overcome fatigue, improve your circulation, calm your nerves, improve sleep, stimulate vital glands and organs, improve your posture, improve your poise, improve your self-confidence. It can eliminate a flabby abdomen, firm a sagging face, strengthen and firm neck muscles, strengthen the lungs, and refresh your mind. Aren't those 15 good reasons for taking time to exercise?

You know some of the effects of exercise even if you don't know what they mean. Run around the block or upstairs and your heart will beat faster and more strongly. During warm-up exercises you usually feel warm and flushed. This is because the blood vessels in your muscles and under your skin are enlarged or dilated. The blood brings more food and oxygen to the muscles and more heat is produced. You usually breathe hard after exercising because, during vigorous exercise, breathing is more rapid, more oxygen is taken in, and more carbon dioxide is exhaled. Exercise usually makes you perspire—water and salt. With regular exercise each individual muscle cell increases in size and the muscles become larger.

Take your time doing exercises. Practice in a quiet place, well ventilated, with fresh air if possible. Wear as little clothing as possible when you exercise. Music can make exercise more enjoyable. Exercising with family or friends can be more fun than exercising alone. But exercise. It will help make your appestat healthy, make you more attractive, and you will feel much more vigorous.

The goal of exercise is physical fitness. Fitness means that your body is functioning properly and that you are well balanced and poised. That involves mind as well as body. The end result is increased joie de vivre. Choose the exercise form you enjoy the most: jogging, fencing, swimming, bicycling, yoga, dancing. Even a person with a heart condition can benefit from dancing, bicycling, and walking. Indeed, victims of heart attacks *should* exercise. Stepped up capacity is the goal, but moderation is the key.

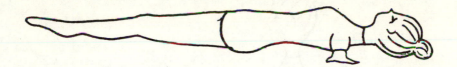

ABDOMINALS

Lie on back with arms outstretched. Sit up slowly and raise knees to chest. Tuck head.

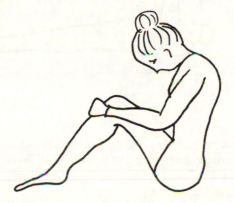

Now extend arms out to sides and legs out in front, keeping them elevated to a count of five.

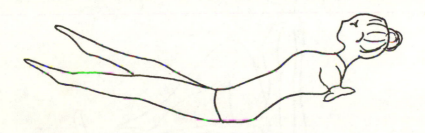

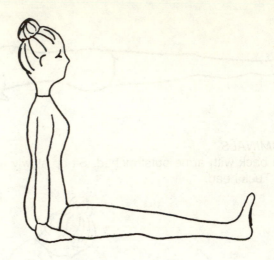

ABDOMINALS

Start in a long sitting position. Raise knee to chest and lower slowly. Alternate legs, keeping back straight throughout exercise.

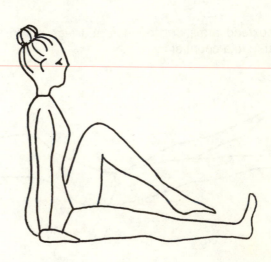

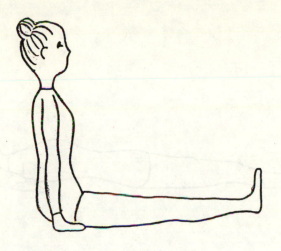

ABDOMINALS

Start in a long sitting position. Raise one leg and lower rapidly. Alternate legs rapidly.

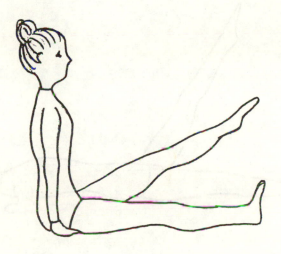

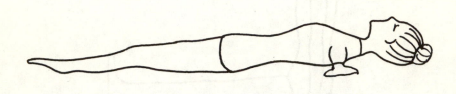

ABDOMINALS
Lie on back on floor with arms outstretched to sides. Raise leg to vertical position then lower slowly to a count of eight.

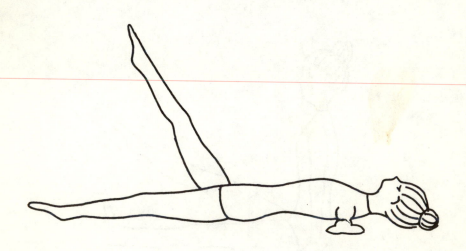

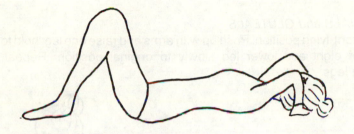

WAIST and ABDOMINALS
Sit ups with knees bent. Touch each elbow to the opposite knee.

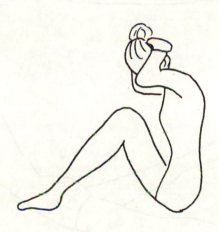

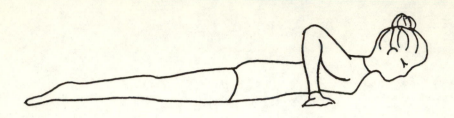

ABDOMINALS and GLUTEALS
Start in a front-lying position. Push up with arms and raise one leg; hold to a count of eight and lower leg slowly to original position. Repeat, alternating legs.

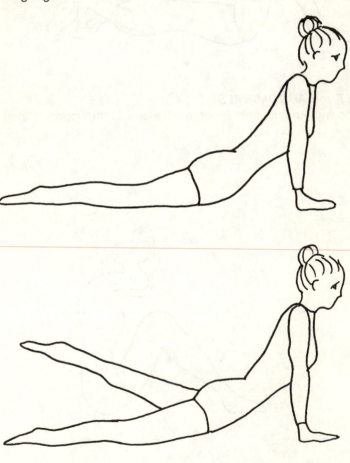

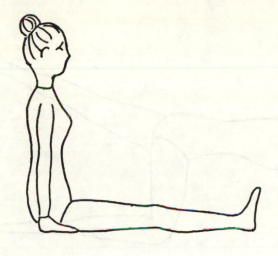

GLUTEALS and ABDOMINALS
Start in long sitting position. Lift hips and arch back. Return to long sitting position. Bring knees up to chest; return legs to original position.

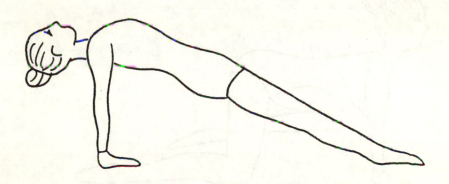

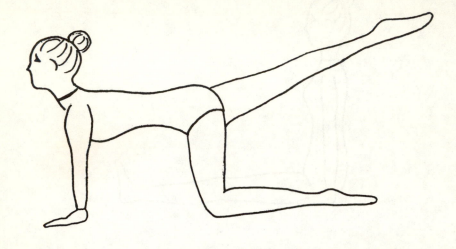

GLUTEALS and THIGHS
Start on all fours. Keep head up and raise leg straight up in back. Bring knee up to chest and extend again. **Repeat with opposite leg.**

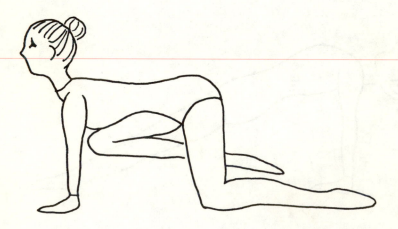

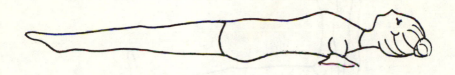

THIGHS and ABDOMINALS
Lie on back with legs straight and arms out to sides. Bend leg, keeping as straight as possible and touch foot to outstretched hand. Repeat exercise, alternating legs.

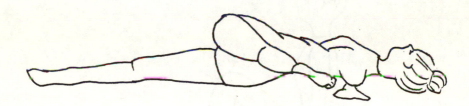

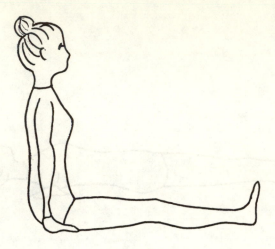

UPPER THIGHS

Start in long sitting position. Bend knee and cross over other leg to touch floor on other side. Repeat with other leg.

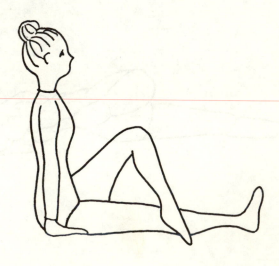

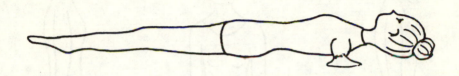

NECK, CHIN and CHEST
Lie on back. Raise head and shoulders off floor and simultaneously pull up slowly with arms. Relax and repeat.

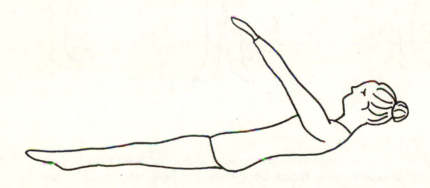

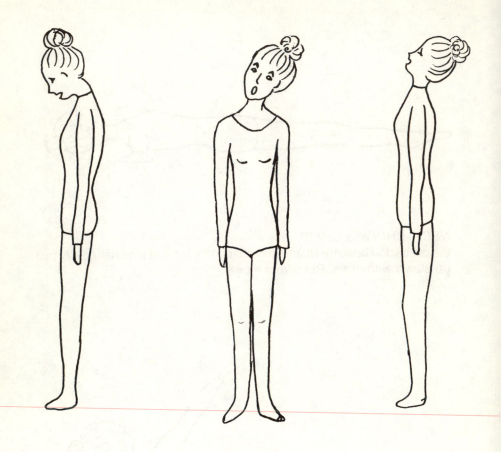

FACE and NECK
Stand erect with hands down at sides. Pull head around to the front, side, back, and other side. Keep rolling head and keep neck muscles taut.

While rotating head, make exaggerated facial contortions—keep mouth wide open, eyebrows arched, and neck muscles taut.

Chapter 11

A Daily Program For a Thinner, Healthier You

ON AWAKENING:

Sip a glass of hot water, preferably mixed with the juice of one-half lemon or one-quarter to one half cup of prune juice.

MEDITATION (15-20 minutes):

Take a comfortable position, sitting in a straight-backed chair or on the floor, or lying on the floor or on your firm-mattressed bed. Consciously relax. Start with the top of your head. Consciously relax the skull. You can't? Well, imagine it relaxing. In time it actually will. Gently move your mind now to your forehead. Relax your forehead. Then your eyes. And the muscles around the eyes. Now the cheeks. The mouth. The chin. The throat. The shoulders. The arms. The fingers. Gently shift the mind back to the torso. Relax the chest. The diaphragm. The waist. The abdomen. The buttocks. The thighs. The legs. The knees. The calves. The ankles. The feet. The toes.

Now you can say a single word to yourself—"love" or "life" or the universal, Eastern-based "om"—gently wiping away intrusive thoughts as they arise in your mind, bringing your mind back to meditation with the mantra—your chosen word.

Or you can concentrate gently on a problem, or planning your day, or prayer. Or you can use Andrew Carnegie's successful method and "meet" with your health and beauty counselors and "discuss" with them the "ideal" you. Discuss with them your program of exercise, your diet, demonstrating the optimistic attitude that is producing this thinner, happier you. *See* yourself at your ideal weight. See yourself at that weight *now*. Picture yourself at your ideal weight—at work, at parties, with friends, with relatives: perhaps dancing, playing tennis, skiing, sailing, doing something you like. Practice seeing yourself at this ideal weight at least five minutes. Chat with your beauty-health counselors: discuss with them any idea you may have: any goal you may have: any need you may feel. Tell them you'll see them soon. Thank them for having spent time with you. Open your eyes.

EXERCISE (15-20 minutes):

Spend a minimum of 15 minutes in different kinds of exercises. including deep breathing—exercises for your ankles, feet, thighs, abdomen, lungs, face, neck, arms, chest. Any problem area. You can perform some of your exercises while lying in bed. You should perform some by an open window, wearing a warm "exercise suit" or long robe or flannelette pajamas or nightgown if the weather is cold. If you are really energetic, you might jog outdoors. A stationary bicycle is a good indoor substitute.

SHOWER OR BATHE:

If you prefer a stimulating shower to a relaxing tub, take a hot one first for two to three minutes, then turn on the cold for 20-30 seconds: then hot, then cold: then hot, then cold. Towel yourself vigorously.

DRESS:

Whether male or female, choose becoming colors. Be sure your clothes are clean and in good repair. Be sure they reflect the ideal you.

BREAKFAST:

Choose your breakfast according to whether you are on a "maintenance" or a reducing diet. If you are pursuing a normal "work life" with no time off for an early-afternoon rest period, choose a minimum of 1000-1200 calories per day if you are female; 1200-1600 calories if male. Remember Larry Paskow's favorite quote: "Breakfast like a king!"

That means protein—egg or chopped meat (lean, good quality), broiled lamb chop, or cottage cheese. Or if you are eating a cereal, a whole-grain one will "stay with you longer." For a change, try millet with milk.

POST-BREAKFAST:

Take vitamin/mineral supplements.

11 a.m.: Vegetable juice (six to eight ounces), or fruit juice mixed 50-50 with water, or "free food" snack such as celery or carrot sticks, or a few slices of raw zucchini or one-half dozen raw mushrooms.

30 MINUTES BEFORE LUNCH:

Six to eight ounces of hot water, with or without lemon juice.

15 MINUTES BEFORE LUNCH:

Walk as briskly as you wish, preferably on the earth or sand. If walking isn't practical for you, practice a few minutes of breathing/stretching exercises, preferably in front of an open window. At the least, just roll your head slowly: forward, to one side, back, to the other side, front, and then reverse. A half-dozen alternating left-to-right, right-to-left "rolls" will relax your neck muscles, your shoulders, and suddenly you'll feel better all over.

LUNCH:

Select any menu from the Harbor Island Spa recommendations that fits within your daily caloric budget. Keep in mind Larry Paskow's admonition: "Lunch like a prince!" That means you can include dessert—a low-calories one. Try to avoid "business lunches." Meet business friends if you wish but try to keep the conversation on subjects that are free of tension—for you digestion's sake. If you must talk business, choose the simplest of foods, most readily digested, and avoid, for your health's sake, anything rich, including sauces, lobster, or anything that you—or nutritionists— find "hard to digest."

POST-LUNCH (if possible):

Relax 10–15 minutes in a quiet place. Relax your body as you did in the morning. You might flood your mind with color—a lovely cool, clear green—green for balance—or a lovely light, or even dark, indigo blue—for peace and relaxation. Now, for a few minutes, idly, gently, easily, picture yourself as the ideal you; visualize yourself as that way *now*.

LATE AFTERNOON:

Low-calorie snack such as one-half grapefruit, or six ounces vegetable juice, or three ounces fruit juice mixed with three ounces water, or a small serving of "diet" gelatin, or a piece of fruit.

PRE-DINNER:

Miditate for 15-20 minutes if you are practicing meditation with a single-word mantra.

Thirty minutes before dinner, drink—sipping it!—six to eight ounces hot water, preferably mixed with the juice of one-half lemon.

A brisk walk or short swim or 15 minutes of other exercise if possible, or a few breathing/stretching exercises.

DINNER:

Choose from the Harbor Island Spa recommendation, or simply enjoy a large mixed green salad with a favorite vegetable-oil dressing, plus, if your calorie allowance permits, a small baked white or sweet potato or yam, and possibly a small serving of cottage cheese, or milk or yogurt.

POST-DINNER:

Take vitamin/mineral supplements, washed down with hot water.

EVENING SNACK:

Six grapes, or one small-to-medium apple or pear, or one-half cantaloupe, or a small slice of other melon or papaya or mango, or one-half banana.

Optional:

Bedtime snack: Diet gelatin, or one-quarter cup of diet yogurt, or herb tea, or artichoke stick.

IN BED, BEFORE SLEEP:

Repeat morning procedure to achieve relaxation.

Counsel with your personally selected Health and Beauty Board—men and women who represent your ideals of health and beauty—living persons or persons from other days or ages, or creations from history, legend, or your own imagination. Talk with them about your successes of the day; gain their counsel and goodwill if you have had failures and did not stay within your caloric ration or failed to exercise; and then, in their presence, with their silent support or verbal encouragement, picture yourself for five minutes *now* at your ideal weight, in optimum health, happy, successful, vibrant, busy!

Picture yourself in attractive, becoming clothes doing exciting or meaningful things, enjoying sports or social activities or anything that fits within your picture of an ideal life. To help you visualize your "Beauty and Health Board," make your selections carefully. Perhaps your Board has only one member, or two or three. It can have as many as five or six, but I don't recommend more than that. See them carefully; use their names when you "talk" with them. Pictures their faces, their bodies, their hair, their clothes. See them as your counselors and also as your peers, as your friends, interested in you, concerned about you, concerned about your health, your success, your happiness. See yourself as one with them; equal— accepted and accepting.

SLEEP:

And happy dreams.

For your health's sake, as well as for your weight-loss goals, try to maintain a *daily* regimen and keep to the caloric ration required to achieve your ideal weight. As you stay with that ration, see your appestat working perfectly, automatically balancing your food intake with your energy output.

If you have a dinner engagement, reduce your caloric intake at breakfast and lunch, but be sure you have some protein and at least a small amount of carbohydrate and fat at all your meals. At dinner, eat freely if this is the day you are "forgetting" your diet, but keep the portions comparatively small and refuse seconds.

If dining out is routine in your life, preplan your menus before you go to a restaurant. If you dine regularly at the homes of friends, let them know you are reducing your caloric intake—make it on doctor's orders, not as if it were simply a whim on your part—or say you are trying to win a bet to lose 30 pounds, or whatever best suits your style, and let your hostesses know that you will *appreciate* their help in keeping you on the straight and narrow. A thoughtful hostess will refrain from serving your favorite cream soup, beef Wellington, or asparagus slathered with hollandaise sauce, plus cherries jubilee or other of what are undoubtedly your favorite foods.

WEEKENDS:

Most of us enjoy a change of routine on weekends, often sleeping later, and sometimes reducing our meals to two hearty ones a day—brunch and supper. For the person who wants to lose weight, this routine represents high-level danger. If your family, or the place where you are visiting, practices the two-meals-a-day program, protect yourself by making your own food program and arm yourself with preplanned snacks or simply arrange to fix yourself small "extra" meals.

Start your days with hot water with lemon or prune juice.

On Saturday or Sunday weigh and measure yourself and record the results. If there is no reduction from the previous Saturday (or Sunday), don't fret about it. Remain optimistic, knowing that a shift in the water balance may be the cause. Stay confident, *knowing* you will show a loss in pounds or inches or both by the succeeding week.

Meditation:

Fifteen to twenty minutes. No more is necessary.

Exercise:

You might extend the time period.

Bathe or shower:

Add a few extras, such as a manicure or pedicure or a facial (if you are a teen-ager or adult, male or female) or shampoo.

Mini-breakfast:

One-half grapefruit, or a small slice of papaya, or one-half banana and a demiserving of cottage cheese or low-calorie yogurt. One cup of herb tea or caffeine-free coffee.

Brunch:

Protein—meat or broiled fish, or lox and bagel, or soft-boiled egg. One slice of toast or small muffin.

Post-brunch:

Take vitamin/mineral supplements.

2 p.m.: Glass of vegetable juice, or fruit-juice-with-water, or piece of fruit.

4:30 p.m.: Herb tea or juice.

5 p.m. (or so): Eat prudently of what the family eats but make sure you have a large raw mixed-green salad, preferably with oil-and-lemon-juice dressing, and, if possible, one cooked yellow vegetable—squash, carrots, sweet potato, yam, or rutabaga.

Post-supper:
Vitamin/mineral supplements.

8 p.m.: Artichoke stick (one) or raw vegetables or diet gelatin.

Bedtime snack:
Four ounces of low-fat milk, if desired. (For hypoglycemics, two ounces of low-fat cheese.)

Sleep-time:
Relaxation, meditation with your Health-and-Beauty Board. Sleep!

Sunday:
Repeat of Saturday, but don't weigh or measure yourself.

To summarize the recommendation, your daily routine should consist of six basic activities or actions:

1) 30 minutes before meals drink hot water, preferably with lemon juice (or prune juice before breakfast).

2) Relax and meditate with your Beauty and Health Board in the morning and the last thing before you sleep.

3) Spead your calorie ration over the three meals plus snack periods, remembering to count any fats or oils used in food preparation within the day's total.

4) Take vitamin/mineral supplements after breakfast and after last meal of the day.

5) Take a minimum of one exercise period a day, or, better, three short ones, or at least some breathing/stretching exercises.

6) Practice an optimistic, confident attitude.

Chapter 12

Menus From Harbor Island Spa

EACH body cell has different requirements so your diet should be varied and balanced in order that each of the millions of cells be provided with the nourishment it requires.

A balanced and varied diet is achieved by choosing from four broad categories of food: the milk group, meat group, vegetables and fruits, breads and cereals.

The milk group includes not only milk but also cheese and other foods made with milk, such as yogurt. The meat group includes fish, poultry, game, and seafood. Vegetarians who eschew meat, poultry, and seafood must obtain their primary protein from milk dishes, eggs, and soybeans and eat enough nuts and vegetables that hopefully the selections will add up to complete protein.

Emphasize variety in selecting fruits and vegetables. A basic rule is to endeavor to have both green and yellow vegetables at least once a day. Experiment with some of the less familiar fruits such as the wonderful papaya, with its blessings for the digestive system, and mango, as well as the more commonly used apples, pears, apricots, and citrus fruits.

''Protein control'' your foods, and view ''seconds'' as an indulgence unnecessary for anyone.

Remember that the health of individual cells depends upon the overall health of the individual. There is an interdependence among the cells, with some acting as ''auxiliaries'' in that, while they themselves are not vital to life, they provide the passage for nourishment for the vital, life-sustaining cells.

Good nutrition is essential to our heart cells, our lungs, our bones, our skin, our hair, our brain, our total life. The single most important thing you can do for your health is to keep in mind that cellular malnutrition is the basis for all malnutrition and that the obese are almost inevitably among our greatest victims of malnutrition.

Remember too that if you drastically restrict your caloric intake, you must sleep and rest more. It will benefit anyone to get the deep rest of meditation twice daily but, if you are on a daily diet of less than 1000 calories, periodic rest, flat on your back on bed or slant board, is essential. It's an error to consume more than one's energy output requires, but it is equal error to consume less.

To step up the 1000-calorie menus that follow to 1200 or 1600, simply increase the size of the servings and/or, instead of making all your snacks nearly calorie-free, or calorie-low, occasionally substitute nuts and seeds as well as fruits.

MENUS—1000 Calories

30 minutes before breakfast:
6-8 ounces hot water, mixed with juice of ½ lemon.

Breakfast:
  Choice of one:
    4 ounces orange, prune, tomato, or grapefruit juice
    or
    ½ grapefruit (no sugar), prunes (3), figs (3), or strawberries (6).

  Choice of one:
    One egg (poached, boiled, or scrambled in Teflon pan)
    or
    3 ounces broiled chopped meat

    or
    ½ cup cottage cheese
    1 slice diet toast
    or
    Special K or Total cereal with 4 ounces skim milk
    or
    ¾ cup oatmeal, farina, Cream of Wheat, buckwheat, or millet with 4 ounces skim milk.

121

MONDAY:

Lunch:
4 oz. tomato juice
6 oz. broiied Sole
Marinated cucumbers
Jello whip (recipe, page 159)
Artichoke Bread Stix

Dinner:
8 oz. roast veal (recipe, page 146)
Hearts of lettuce and tomato
½ cup string beans (recipe, page 154)
Melon—2″ wedge
Artichoke Bread Stix

TUESDAY:

Lunch:
Chef's Salad bowl (recipe, page 130)
Chocolate mousse (recipe, page 160)
Artichoke Bread Stix

Dinner:
⅔ cup broth
8 oz. chopped steak
½ cup carrots
Asparagus salad (recipe, page 129)
Baked fresh peaches (recipe, page 159)
Artichoke Bread Stix

WEDNESDAY:

Lunch:
4 oz. cranberry juice
Tuna salad platter
Baked apricot whip (recipe, page 158)
Artichoke Bread Stix

Dinner:
½ broiled chicken
½ cup Brussels sprouts
Tossed green salad
½ grapefruit
Artichoke Bread Stix

THURSDAY:

Lunch:
Shrimp platter
Pineapple ice cream (recipe, page 161)
Artichoke Bread Stix

Dinner:
⅔ cup vegetable soup (recipe, page 128)
Baby flounder (recipe, page 138)
½ cup stewed tomatoes
Hearts lettuce and cucumber
Fruit compote (recipe, page 201)
Artichoke Bread Stix

122

FRIDAY:

Lunch:
4 oz. V-8 juice
Chicken salad platter (recipe, page 131)
Coconut mousse (recipe, page 160)
Artichoke Bread Stix

Dinner:
8 oz. broiled salmon
½ cup spinach
Mixed green salad
Baked Apple (recipe, page 158)
Artichoke Bread Stix

SATURDAY:

Lunch:
Mushroom omelette (recipe, page 137)
Marinated cucumbers
½ cantaloupe
Artichoke Bread Stix

Dinner:
Shrimp cocktail (3 shrimp)
8 oz. sirloin steak
Baked acorn squash (recipe, page 155)
Tossed salad
Jello cake (recipe, page 159)
Artichoke Bread Stix

SUNDAY:

Lunch:
4 oz. Nova Scotia lox (recipe, page 139)
with cream cheese and bagel
2 slices tomato
Strawberry Bavarian (recipe, page 161)

Dinner:
4 oz. tomato juice
8 oz. roast beef
3 spears broccoli
Sliced tomato
½ cup sliced peaches
Artichoke Bread Stix

****

SAMPLE BREAKFASTS:

1 small sliced orange	4 oz. tomato juice	½ sliced banana
1 scrambled egg	5/8 oz. Total cereal	or 4 oz. prune juice
1 slice diet toast	4 oz. skim milk	2 egg whites scrambled in Teflon pan
Hot beverage	Hot beverage	2 oz. diet cottage cheese
		1 slice diet toast
		Hot beverage

SAMPLE LUNCHES:

Tuna salad platter	6 oz. broiled sole	4 oz. chopped steak
4 Artichoke Bread Stix	Tossed salad, 2 oz.	½ cup chopped lettuce
Jello whip (recipe,	vinaigrette dressing	½ cup marinated
page 159)	4 Bread Stix	green beans
Hot beverage	2 slices unsweetened	Coffee mousse (recipe
	pineapple	page 160)
	Hot beverage	4 Bread Stix
		Hot beverage

SAMPLE DINNERS:

½ Bar-B-Q chicken	6 oz. lean roast beef	2 lean baby lamb
(recipe, page 148)	½ cup carrots	chops
3 asparagus spears	½ cup marinated	¼ cup acorn squash
1 cup chopped lettuce	cucumbers	Tossed green salad
2 slices tomato	Artichoke Bread Stix	2 oz. dressing
½ grapefruit	Pineapple ice cream	1 baked peach
4 Artichoke Bread Stix	(recipe, page 161)	(recipe, page 159)
Hot beverage	Hot beverage	4 Bread Stix
		Hot beverage

*****

124

MENUS— 600 Calories

SAMPLE BREAKFASTS:

4 oz. orange juice	½ grapefruit	3 prunes
1 poached egg	1 box Special K	½ slice diet toast
½ slice diet toast	4 oz. skim milk	2 oz. diet cottage
Hot beverage	Hot beverage	cheese
		1 teaspoon diet jelly
		Hot beverage

SAMPLE LUNCHES:

Shrimp platter, garni	4 oz. broiled sole	Chef's salad
Jello whip	½ cup marinated	(recipe page 130)
4 Bread Stix	zucchini	2 oz. french
Hot beverage	4 Bread Stix	dressing
	½ cup blueberries	4 Bread Stix
	Hot beverage	Jello cake (recipe,
		page 159)
		Hot beverage

SAMPLE DINNERS:

6 oz. chopped steak	6 oz. broiled chicken	6 oz. roast veal
3 broccoli spears	½ cup green beans	½ cup stewed
Lettuce with tomato	Mixed green salad	tomatoes
slices	2 oz. vinaigrette	½ cup salt-free cole
Bread Stix	dressing (recipe, page	slaw (recipe, page
¼ cantaloupe	166)	131)
	Bread Stix	½ cup strawberries
	Coconut mousse	Bread Stix
	(recipe, page 160)	Hot beverage
	Hot beverage	

****

125

Chapter 13

Harbor Island Spa Cookbook

WE have three credos about food at Harbor Island Spa. It should be good for our (individual) bodies, delicious to taste, and attractive to look at. While we will serve baked potatoes with sour cream or butter to nondieters, as well as wine, highballs, and nondietetic cakes and rolls and breads, the Harbor Island Spa recipes listed here are designed to reduce weight and control it, to reduce cholesterol levels, and to restrict salt intake. Therefore the recipes specify artificial sweetener instead of sugar, arrow root instead of flour for thickening,* artichoke-breadstick crumbs for breading, Vege-Sal instead of salt, and almost always polyunsaturated vegetable oils.

The number of calories that follows each recipe title is the calorie value *per serving* (unless otherwise stated), according to the number of servings given at the end of the recipe. Should you wish to increase the portion size to increase the day's total caloric intake (perhaps from 1200 to 1600 for an active person on a maintenance diet), multiply the calories per serving by the number of servings for the total caloric value of the recipe. Then divide the total calories by the new number of desired servings for the value of each new larger serving.

---

* 1 teaspoon arrowroot equals 1 tablespoon flour

2 teaspoons arrowroot equal 1 tablespoon cornstarch

SOUPS

CREAM OF MUSHROOM (60 calories)
2 cups skim milk
2 tablespoons arrowroot
4 tablespoons polyunsaturated oil
¼ teaspoon Vege-Sal
½ cup fresh mushrooms, sliced

    In a saucepan, heat 2 teaspoons oil. Add mushrooms and Vege-Sal. Saute lightly. Heat remaining oil in separate saucepan over low heat. Blend in arrowroot. Add milk slowly to arrowroot, blending well, and heat slowly, stirring constantly until mixture thickens. Add mushrooms. Simmer, covered, 30 minutes. 4 servings.

LENTIL (75 calories)
1½ cups dried lentils
6 cups water
1 tablespoon polyunsaturated oil
1 teaspoon Vege-Sal
1 tablespoon arrowroot
1 medium onion, diced

    Wash lentils and soak overnight. Heat oil in deep pot. Stir in arrowroot. Add other ingredients, including water in which lentils were soaked. Cover and cook until lentils are soft (about 90 minutes). 6 servings.

FRENCH ONION (75 calories)
4 onions sliced very thin
2 tablespoons polyunsaturated oil
4 cups water
2 oz. sauterne
few drops Maggi or Kitchen Bouquet
Vege-Sal to taste
pepper
grated Parmesan cheese

    Saute onions in oil until onions are transparent. Add water and wine. Simmer, covered, 15 minutes. Add Maggi or Kitchen Bouquet, Vege-Sal, and pepper. Blend thoroughly. Serve in individual bowls with cheese sprinkled on top or pass cheese separately. 4 servings.

CHICKEN BROTH (50 calories per cup, not including garnish))
8 chicken wings, washed
1/8 cup celery, chopped
1 medium-size onion, quartered
1 bay leaf
¾ teaspoon Vege-Sal
¼ teaspoon white pepper
4 cups water
   Put all ingredients in pot. Cook, covered, for about 2 hours, until meat possibly falls off bones. Remove meat and bones and reserve meat for later use in chicken salad or other dish. Simmer soup, covered, over low heat for 30 minutes longer. Strain broth, then refrigerate. When fat comes to top, skim off fat. Before serving, put skimmed broth in pot, drop in any desired accompaniment (farfel, mandlen, dumplings, etc.) and reheat 6-8 servings.

VEGETABLE (75 calories)
1 lb. boneless chuck, cubed
1 soup bone, cracked
4 cups water
2 teaspoons Vege-Sal
2 cups canned tomatoes (use salt-free in sodium-restricted diets)
½ cup diced carrots
½ cup diced celery
1 tablespoon parsley, minced
1 small onion, diced
   Place chuck and soup bone in kettle with water and Vege-Sal. Cover, and bring to boil. Add remaining ingredients and stir. Reduce heat. Simmer, covered, for about 1 hour. Cool, then refrigerate. When fat rises, skim fat before reheating to serve. 6 servings.

SALADS

ASPARAGUS (15 calories)
4 chilled asparagus spears (canned, white, salt-free)
chopped lettuce
2 pimento strips

Place asparagus on chopped lettuce with pimento strips. Serve with vinaigrette dressing (recipe, page 166). 1 serving.

AVOCADO (95 calories)
1 large avocado
2 cups chopped fresh tomatoes
1 small onion, finely chopped
⅓ cup diet cottage cheese
3 tablespoons polyunsaturated oil
1 tablespoon lemon juice
1 teaspoon Vege-Sal
pepper

Peel avocado, remove seed, and chop coarsely. Toss with remaining ingredients in a chilled salad bowl until thoroughly combined with oil and seasonings. Cover bowl and chill in refrigerator for 15–30 minutes before serving. 4 main-course servings.

BEAN (25 calories)
2 cups cooked green string beans (canned, fresh, or frozen)
⅔ cup white vinegar
⅓ cup water
1 packet Sweet'n Low or equivalent substitute
¼ cup (total) chopped green pepper, pimento, and scallion

Combine all ingredients except beans. Blend. Add beans and blend well. Chill in refrigerator 2 or more hours. 4 servings.

129

CABBAGE AND BANANA (41 calories)
2 cups shredded cabbage (chilled)
1 banana, sliced
½ cup Balanaise mayonnaise
⅓ teaspoon Vege-Sal
    Combine ingredients. Mix thoroughly. 4 servings.

CANTALOUPE WITH DIET COTTAGE CHEESE (125 calories)
    Cut cantaloupe in half. Remove seeds. Fill each half with diet cottage cheese. Chill (about 10 minutes) and serve. 2 main-course servings.

CARROT COLE SLAW (25 calories)
3 cups white cabbage, chilled and shredded
2 carrots, grated
½ green pepper, chopped very fine
1 teaspoon Vege-Sal
¼ teaspoon pepper
1 packet Sweet'n Low or equivalent substitute
1 teaspoon garlic powder
¼ cup white vinegar
4 tablespoons Balanaise mayonnaise
    Turn shredded cabbage into chilled salad bowl. add carrots and green pepper. Blend. Mix seasonings, sweetener, and vinegar. Blend into mayonnaise. Pour over salad and toss until well mixed. Cover salad bowl and chill until ready to serve. 6 servings.

CHEF'S SALAD BOWL, JULIENNE (175 calories)
1 medium head iceberg lettuce, washed and dried
4 ounces julienne turkey
4 ounces julienne skim-milk mozzarella cheese
2 whole tomatoes
½ medium-size cucumber
2 pepper rings
    Break or cut lettuce into bite-size portions. Divide into two chilled individual serving bowls. Divide turkey and cheese between the bowls. Wash and dry tomatoes and cut each into four parts. Ring each bowl with one quartered tomato. Garnish with pepper ring. Chill. Serve with French dressing (recipe, page 165). 2 main-course servings.

CHICKEN, GARNI (or TURKEY) (225 calories)

4 cups cooked chicken chunks (or turkey)
1 cup diced celery
1 cup diced green pepper
1 cup Balanaise mayonnaise
1 teaspoon Vege-Sal
⅛ teaspoon pepper
lettuce leaves
garnish: sliced cucumber, sliced tomato

    Place first six items in chilled bowl and toss until chicken is well blended with other ingredients. Refrigerate until cold. Serve on lettuce leaves garnished with tomato and cucumber. 4 main-course servings.

COLE SLAW (approximately 25 calories)

2 cups cabbage, chilled and shredded
1 sweet red pepper, finely chopped
1 cup white vinegar
1 cup unsweetened pineapple juice
1 package Sweet'n Low or equivalent substitute

    Combine vinegar, juice, and sweetener. Mix well. Add cabbage and red pepper. Blend thoroughly. 4-6 servings.

CRAB MEAT (225 calories)

1 lb. cooked crabmeat
¼ cup diced celery
¼ cup diced green pepper
¼ teaspoon Vege-Sal
½ cup Balanaise mayonnaise
crisp lettuce
2 tomatoes, sliced
2 hard-cooked eggs, sliced

    Combine crabmeat, celery, and green pepper in chilled bowl. Mix mayonnaise and Vege-Sal. Toss well with crabmeat mixture. Spoon over lettuce in six individual serving bowls. Garnish with tomato and egg slices. Chill. 6 main-course servings.

CUCUMBER (½ cup, 18 calories)
4 medium cucumbers
¼ cup white vinegar
½ packet Sweet'n Low or equivalent substitute
2 tablespoons diced green pepper
strips of pimento
    Cut off points of cucumbers and pare. Slice crosswise into thin slices. Sprinkle with sweetener. Add green pepper and pimento strips. Pour vinegar over mixture and toss well. Chill. 6 servings.

FRUIT PLATTER WITH DIET COTTAGE CHEESE (175 calories)
2 pear halves packed in water (canned)
2 peach halves packed in water (canned)
¼ apple, sliced
¼ orange, sliced
½ cup diet cottage cheese
lettuce, broken into bite sizes or half leaves
    Arrange lettuce on two chilled serving plates. Place cottage cheese in center. Alternate fruit around cheese. Chill before serving. 2 main-course servings.

MELON MOLD (approximately 14 calories)
1 package lime-flavored gelatin
1 pint hot water
1½ cups melon balls
lettuce
    Dissolve gelatin in hot water. Chill. When slightly thickened, fold in melon balls. Turn into mold and chill until firm. Unmold on crisp lettuce. 6 servings.

SARDINE PLATTER GARNI (175 calories)
1 3¾ oz. can water-packed sardines, drained (skinless and boneless)
1 slice Spanish onion
2 slices tomato
2 slices cucumber
1 sprig parsley
2 lettuce leaves
    Place lettuce on chilled plate. In center, place sardines. Garnish with other ingredients. 1 main-course serving.

SEAFOOD (175 calories)
1 lb. mixed seafood (cooked shrimp, sole, flounder, other)
1 cup Balanaise mayonnaise
½ cup chopped celery
½ cup chopped green pepper
2 teaspoons Vege-Sal
lettuce leaves
tomato slices, cucumber slices, lemon wedges as garnish

Cut or break fish into fairly small pieces. Combine mayonnaise, celery, green pepper, and Vege-Sal and add to the fish, mixing well. Serve on lettuce leaves, garnished with tomato, cucumber, and lemon. 4 main-course servings.

SPRING (80 calories)
1 cup diet cottage cheese
2 cups (total) chopped vegetables:
     cucumber
     tomato
     green pepper
     radishes
     chives or scallions
lettuce leaves (2)

Divide lettuce between two chilled salad plates. Put ½ cup cottage cheese into center of each leaf. Arrange chopped vegetables, which have been mixed together, or kept separate, as desired, around cheese. Chill before serving. 2 main-course servings.

TOMATO ASPIC (76 calories)
1½ envelopes Knox unflavored gelatin
3 cups V-8 juice
juice, ½ lemon
dash Vege-Sal
dash pepper
2 drops Worcestershire Sauce
¼ cup (total) chopped onion and chopped celery

Soften gelatin in cup of vegetable juice and stir until dissolved. Bring remaining juice to boil. Add other ingredients. Simmer about 10 minutes. Strain out vegetables, saving juice. Combine juice and softened gelatin. Stir well and pour into mold. Chill until firm. 5 servings.

TOMATO SURPRISE (175 calories)
1 can (7½ oz.) water-packed tuna
½ cup diced celery
½ cup diced green pepper
dash Vege-Sal
½ cup Balanaise mayonnaise
lettuce leaves

   Combine tuna, broken into flakes, with celery, pepper, Vege-Sal. Blend in mayonnaise. Chill. Arrange lettuce leaves on chilled platter to form cups. Fill each lettuce cup with tuna salad. 2 main-course servings.

EGG DISHES

FLUFFY OMELETTE WITH DIET COTTAGE CHEESE (90 calories)
1 tablespoon polyunsaturated oil
2 eggs
2 tablespoons water
1 teaspoon Vege-Sal
½ cup diet cottage cheese
    Heat oil in skillet or omelette pan over low, low heat. Beat eggs, Vege-Sal, and water until barely blended. Pour into pan. Slide pan back and forth rapidly over heat only long enough to brown bottom of eggs. Place cottage cheese on half of the omelette opposite handle of pan. Loosen edge of omelette with spatula. Fold unfilled omelette half over to cover cottage cheese. Tilt pan. Slide omelette out onto warm plate. 2 servings.

SPANISH OMELETTE (140 calories)
1 cup stewed tomatoes (canned or fresh)
¼ cup diced green pepper
1 tablespoon polyunsaturated oil
¼ cup diced onion
¼ cup diced celery
½ cup sliced mushrooms
    Place tomatoes in sauce pan and heat. Heat oil in skillet. Add vegetables and saute until browned. Add to tomatoes and simmer. Use as filling for 3-egg FLUFFY OMELETTE.

3-EGG FLUFFY OMELETTE (95 calories)
(no oil; use Teflon pan)
3 eggs
3 tablespoons water
½ teaspoon Vege-Sal
    Beat ingredients together until barely blended. Follow directions for FLUFFY OMELETTE above. Use SPANISH OMELETTE mixture for filling instead of diet cottage cheese. 3 servings (235 calories per serving for Spanish Omelette.)

135

CURRIED AVOCADO OMELETTE (195 calories)

6 eggs, separated
½ teaspoon Vege-Sal
¼ teaspoon white pepper
2 teaspoons curry powder
2 tablespoons polyunsaturated oil
1 cup cubed avocado
watercress garnish

Beat egg yolks. Beat egg whites until soft peaks form. Blend seasonings into whites. Fold yolks into whites. Heat oil in pan. Drop in egg mixture. When bottom is lightly browned and omelette is beginning to set, place avocado cubes on half of omelette opposite beginning to set, place avocado cubes on half of omelette opposite handle of pan. Loosen edges of omelette. Fold empty half of omelette over to cover avocado. Tilt pan and slide on heated platter. Garnish with watercress. 6 servings.

BAKED EGGS WITH SWISS CHEESE (150 calories)

1 tablespoon polyunsaturated oil
3 oz. Swiss cheese, grated, and
⅓ cup Swiss cheese, grated
6 eggs
1 teaspoon Vege-Sal
1/8 teaspoon white pepper
1 tablespoon parsley, finely chopped
1 tablespoon chives, finely chopped
1 tablespoon onion finely chopped
1 tablespoon chervil, finely chopped (optional)
1 tablespoon sweet butter

Preheat oven at 350–375 degrees. Oil earthenware baking dish. Sprinkle over it 3 ounces Swiss cheese, grated. Break eggs over cheese, taking care not to break yolks. Sprinkle with Vege-Sal and pepper. Mix remaining Swiss cheese with parsley, chives, onion, and chervil. Scatter over eggs. Top with bits of butter. Bake 10–12 minutes until top bubbles and is browned. Serve at once. 6 servings. Note: instead of large earthenware dish, oiled individual ramekins may be used.

MUSHROOM OMELETTE (160 calories)

2 tablespoons polyunsaturated oil
1 cup diced mushrooms
2 eggs
2 tablespoons water
1 teaspoon Vege-Sal

Heat 1 tablespoon oil in skillet and add diced mushrooms. Saute until just brown, then remove from heat. Beat eggs, water, and seasoning lightly. Heat other tablespoon oil in omelette pan over low heat. Pour egg mixture into omelette pan. Slide pan back and forth over heat until bottom of omelette is barely brown. Place mushrooms on half of omelette opposite the handle of the pan and loosen edge of uncovered half of omelette with a spatula. Fold over plain-egg half of omelette, tilt pan, and slide out onto a warm plate. 2 servings.

FISH AND SEAFOOD

BAKED BASS (260 calories)
2 lbs. bass (cleaned)
¼ cup polyunsaturated oil
1 small onion, minced
1 tablespoon Worcestershire Sauce
juice, 1 orange
juice, ½ lemon
Vege-Sal and pepper

Preheat oven to 400 degrees. Rub oil on fish. Rub seasonings and onion on fish. Place fish on rack in flat baking dish or pan. Pour Worcestershire Sauce and juices over fish. Cover bottom of pan with half-inch water. (Never let pan or baking dish become dry.) Bake at 400 degrees for 10 minutes per pound or until fish flakes with fork. Baste fish often with water and juices from bottom of pan. If fish starts to become too brown, cover top of baking dish loosely with foil. 4 servings.

BROILED BABY FLOUNDER (175 calories)
2 lbs. whole fish (dressed)
polyunsaturated oil
paprika
lemon parsley sauce (recipe, page xxx)

Place fish in broiling pan. Brush with oil and sprinkle with paprika. Broil until fish flakes easily with fork but is still moist. Serve with lemon parsley sauce. 4 servings.

FILET OF FLOUNDER ALMONDINE (165 calories)
2 lbs. filet of flounder
⅓ cup polyunsaturated oil
paprika
¼ cup slivered almonds
parsley
lemon wedges

Brush fish lightly with oil. Sprinkle with paprika. Broil until fish flakes easily with fork and is well browned. Put remaining oil in saucepan. Heat. Brown almonds lightly in oil. Place fish on heated

138

serving platter. Garnish with browned almonds. Ring fish with lemon wedges and parsley. 4 servings.

GEFILTÉ FISH (150 calories)
1 lb. (total) cooked filet of pike and sole
2 eggs, separated
1 small onion, grated
½ teaspoon white pepper
2 teaspoons Vege-Sal
1 tablespoon polyunsaturated oil
2 tablespoons matzo meal
½ cup water

Chop fish fine and place in bowl. Beat egg yolks well. Add onion, seasonings, oil, matzo meal, and water. Beat. Add to fish and mix thoroughly. Beat egg whites until stiff but not dry. Slowly fold into fish mixture. Moisten hands with water and form mixture into balls. Put aside while making stock.

STOCK
2 onions, diced
2 carrots, sliced
1 stalk celery, chopped
1/8 teaspoon pepper
2 cups water
1 teaspoon Knox unflavored gelatin

Put all ingredients except gelatin into pot. Bring to a boil. Lower flame. Carefully place fish balls into simmering stock. Cover pot and cook over low heat one hour. Remove fish balls and place in shallow serving dish. Strain stock and add gelatin to stock. Stir until gelatin is dissolved. Pour stock over fish balls. Chill until firm. 5 servings.

NOVA SCOTIA LOX, TOASTED BAGEL (360 calories)
4 oz. Nova Scotia lox
1 oz. cream cheese
2 slices tomato
lettuce leaves
toasted water bagel

Place lettuce on plate. Arrange lox on lettuce. Arrange cream cheese and sliced tomato around lox. Serve with hot toasted bagel. 1 serving.

SALMON IN ASPIC (450 calories)
4 lbs. fresh salmon cut into 8 oz. portions.
Salmon stock
    Save head, tail, and any leftover pieces of salmon for stock.

STOCK
salmon head and other salmon leftovers
2½ quarts cold water
1 quart white vinegar
1 cup lemon juice
¼ cup Sweet'n Low or equivalent substitute
1 medium onion, chopped
2 whole carrots
2 celery stalks
¼ cup dried pickling spices (tied in cheese cloth)
4 envelopes Knox unflavored gelatin
    Bring all ingredients except gelatin to full boil and boil 20 minutes. Lower flame. Simmer 40 minutes. Strain and place clear broth in deep pot. Lower salmon steaks into broth carefully. (Be sure broth covers salmon. Add water if broth is insufficient.) Cover. Cook until salmon turns pink and comes to top of pot (approximately 25 minutes). Remove salmon to shallow serving dish. Add gelatin to broth and stir until dissolved. Pour stock/gelatine mixture over salmon steaks to depth of about ½ inch. Refrigerate until firm. 8 servings.

BROILED SCALLOPS (140 calories)
2 lbs. baby scallops
1/8 cup polyunsaturated oil
paprika
garlic powder
lemon wedges
    Place scallops on broiler pan. Brush with oil Sprinkle with paprika and garlic powder. Broil until golden brown. Serve with lemon wedges. 8 servings.

SHRIMP CREOLE (70 calories)
1 cup cooked shrimp
1 tablespoon polyunsaturated oil
½ cup onion, chopped
½ cup green pepper, chopped
¼ clove garlic, minced
1/8 teaspoon paprika
1 cup stewed tomatoes (canned or fresh)
pepper

Heat oil in saucepan. Add onion, green pepper, garlic, and paprika. Saute gently until pepper is tender, stirring frequently. Add tomatoes and dash of pepper. Boil gently 5 minutes. Add shrimp and simmer 10 minutes. 4 servings.

MEAT

BRAISED BEEF (450 calories)
4 lbs. brisket of beef
2 tablespoons polyunsaturated oil
1/8 teaspoon pepper
½ cup diced celery
½ cup diced turnip
½ cup diced onion
1 tablespoon chopped parsley
½ bay leaf
2 tablespoons arrowroot
2 cups boiling water

Heat oil in heavy skillet. Pepper meat and brown in skillet on all sides. Surround meat with vegetables. Add water and cover skillet tightly. Simmer slowly about 3½ hours. If possible, refrigerate overnight for fat to rise, then remove fat. Reheat when ready to serve, and place meat on heated platter. Drain vegetables and place around meat. Thicken liquid in skillet with arrowroot. Pass gravy in separate serving dish. 8 servings.

BRISKET OF BEEF (255 Calories)
Marinade (recipe, page **166**)
3 lbs. beef brisket
½ cup sliced onion
½ cup sliced carrots
½ cup diced celery, including leaves
1 teaspoon Vege-Sal
hot water

Marinate beef overnight. Put beef in deep pot and cover with hot water. Add vegetables and cover pot. Simmer gently about 40 minutes until meat is tender (do not boil). Add Vege-Sal when half done. Add more water if necessary. If possible, refrigerate overnight for fat to rise, then skim fat. Reheat when ready to serve and serve with horseradish sauce. Six 4-ounce servings.

BROCHETTE OF SIRLOIN TIPS (250 calories)

2 lbs. boned sirloin steak
2 onions, sliced
2 tomatoes, cut in wedges
½ lb. mushroom caps
2 tablespoons polyunsaturated oil
½ teaspoon Vege-Sal
¼ teaspoon pepper
¼ teaspoon garlic powder
6 metal skewers

Cut sirloin into 1 inch cubes. Alternate beef, onion, tomato wedges, and mushroom caps on metal skewers. In bowl, stir together oil and seasonings. Brush mixture over items on skewers. Let stand about one hour, brushing meat/vegetable mixture with marinade periodically until all marinade is used. Broil about 3 inches from source of heat for about 10 minutes, turning occasionally to brown evenly. 6 servings.

BROILED LIVER (260 Calories)

1½ lbs. liver
2 tablespoons polyunsaturated oil
1 teaspoon Vege-Sal
¼ teaspoon pepper
lemon juice

Brush liver with oil. Broil at high heat approximately 6 minutes, turning often. Remove from broiler to heated serving platter. Sprinkle with seasonings and a few drops of lemon juice. Six 4-ounce servings.

CHOPPED BEEF PATTIES (225 calories)

2 lbs. lean ground chuck
3 oz. tomato juice
3 oz. water
1 teaspoon Vege-Sal

Combine juice, water, and seasoning. Pour over ground chuck. Mix thoroughly and shape into patties. Chill ½ hour. Broil. 6 servings.

143

BOILED CORNED BEEF (250 calories)
3 lbs. corned beef
¼ cup dried pickling spices
water to cover beef

Place meat in skillet. Add spices. Cover with cold water. Simmer until meat is tender (about 1½–2 hours). 6 servings.

MEAT LOAF WITH SAUCE (250 calories)
2 lbs. chuck, ground
2 eggs
1 cup bread stix crumbs
1 teaspoon Vege-Sal
½ teaspoon pepper

Preheat oven to 350 degrees. In large bowl, beat eggs slightly. Mix in chuck, then crumbs and seasonings. Combine lightly (meat will be juicier if you handle it as little as possible). Shape in oval loaf and place in baking dish. Bake 50 minutes, basting at start of cooking and periodically thereafter with:

MEAT LOAF SAUCE
½ cup salt-free catsup
1 tablespoon Worcestershire Sauce
⅓ cup white vinegar
1 tablespoon chili powder
2 tablespoons chopped onion

Mix all ingredients together in bowl. Use to baste meat loaf. 8 servings.

SPICED POT ROAST (240 calories)
2½ lbs. rump pot roast
1 small onion, sliced
1 bay leaf
½ teaspoon whole peppercorns
Vege-Sal and ground pepper
½ cup white vinegar
½ cup water

Rub meat thoroughly with Vege-Sal and ground pepper. Put in kettle. Add onion, bay leaf, and peppercorns. Mix vinegar and water and pour over meat. Let stand overnight. Heat oven to 400 degrees.

144

Place meat in roasting pan and sear in oven until browned. Reduce heat to 325–350 degrees. cover pan and cook until meat is tender (about 1½ hours). 4 servings.

PRIME RIBS OF BEEF (4 oz., 145 calories)
6-8 lbs. rolled prime ribs of beef
oil
garlic powder
pepper
Preheat oven to 350 degrees. Rub garlic powder and pepper into beef. Place beef on rach in roasting pan. roast 20–30 minutes per pound, depending upon degree of rareness desired. Let stand 15 minutes before slicing. 8–10 servings.

BROILED SIRLOIN STEAK WITH MUSHROOM CAPS (450 calories)
four 8-oz. lean sirloin steaks
Vege-Sal
2 tablespoons polyunsaturated oil
1 cup mushroom caps
Sprinkle steak with Vege-Sal. Place on broiler rack and broil to desired degree of doneness. While broiling (approximately 5–8 minutes for each side), heat oil in skillet and saute mushroom caps, stirring frequently. Serve steak garnished with mushrooms. 4 servings.

TERIYAKI STEAK (245 calories)
Marinade (recipe, page **166**)
3 lbs. lean beef shoulder, cut thin (as for London broil)
Pierce steak with fork. Put in bowl with marinade. Refrigerate overnight or longer, turning periodically. Broil five minutes on either side. 6 servings.

BARBECUED VEAL CHOPS (260 calories)
4 tablespoons polyunsaturated oil
4 lean veal chops
3 tablespoons soy sauce
3 tablespoons catsup
1 tablespoon vinegar
½ packet Sweet'n Low or equivalent substitute
¼ teaspoon pepper
1 clove garlic, minced

    Heat oil in skillet. Add veal chops and brown slowly on each side. Combine remaining ingredients in bowl Pour over veal chops and cover skillet. Cook slowly until chops are tender (about 30–35 minutes). 4 servings.

RAGOUT OF VEAL (235 calories)
1 tablespoon polyunsaturated oil
3 onions, finely chopped
3 tomatoes, sliced
2 lbs. veal
2 carrots, diced
2 tablespoons parsley, chopped
1 packet Sweet'n Low or equivalent substitute
1 teaspoon Vege-Sal
¼ teaspoon pepper
1 cup canned stewed tomatoes

    Heat oil in skillet. Add onions and saute until transparent. Add sliced tomatoes. Wash veal and put in pan wet. Add all other ingredients. Cover skillet and stew slowly 2 hours. Six 4-oz. servings.

ROAST SHOULDER OF VEAL (245 calories)
4 lbs. lean veal, rolled
1 medium onion, sliced
2 stalks celery, diced
2 carrots, sliced into rounds
½ teaspoon pepper
1 teaspoon Vege-Sal

    Preheat oven to 350 degrees. Rub roast with pepper and Vege-Sal. Place roast in shallow roasting pan and add onion, celery, and carrots. Do not cover. Roast about 1½ hours. 8 servings.

VEAL PAPRIKA WITH DIET NOODLES (235 calories)

1½ lbs. veal steak, cubed
2 tablespoons polyunsaturated oil
2 tablespoons chopped onion
1 teaspoon paprika
½ cup diet sour cream
DeBoles diet noodles

Heat oil in skillet. Add veal, onions, and paprika. Saute until browned. When veal is soft (about 10 minutes), add sour cream. Cover and cook over low heat about 25 minutes. Serve with DeBoles diet noodles (see resource list, page   205). 6 servings.

ROAST LEG OF LAMB WITH MINT SAUCE (325 calories)

3-pound leg of lamb
¼ teaspoon pepper
1 teaspoon Vege-Sal
mint sauce (recipe, page   164)

Preheat oven to 300 degrees. Sprinkle pepper and Vege-Sal over lamb. Place on rack in open roasting pan. Bake until lamb is cooked to desired degree of doneness, allowing 22-25 minutes per pound. While cooking, baste periodically with mint sauce. Four 4-ounce servings.

POULTRY

BAR-B-Q-CHICKEN (250 calories)
1 14-oz. bottle diet catsup
½ small can unsweetened pineapple juice
3 drops Tabasco Sauce
3 drops Soy Sauce
2 packages Sweet'n Low or equivalent substitute
roasting chicken (3–3½ pounds)
juice 1 lemon
1 teaspoon Vege-Sal
1 clove garlic

Blend first five ingredients in sauce pan. Simmer one hour. Preheat oven to 350 degrees. Wipe chicken inside and out with damp paper towel. Sliver one end of garlic clove. Rub chicken cavity with garlic, then sprinkle with half of mixed lemon juice and Vege-Sal. Repeat process on outside of chicken. Roast chicken on wire rack in open roasting pan for 40 minutes. Remove from oven. Pierce chicken in several places with fork. Baste with Bar-B-Q-sauce. Roast 20 minutes longer. 8 servings.

CHICKEN CACCIATORA (200 calories)
2½ pound chicken, cut into 8 pieces
1 16-oz. can tomatoes
1 small onion, chopped
1 clove garlic, minced
1 bay leaf
1 teaspoon Vege-Sal
2 cups water

Put chicken into pot with 2 cups cold water. Heat water to boiling, then reduce heat. Cover and simmer 20 minutes. Mash tomatoes to pulp and put into pot with chicken. Add onion, garlic, bay leaf, and Vege-Sal. Cover and simmer 30 minutes longer. 6 servings.

CHICKEN SAUTE WITH VEGETABLES (250 calories)

1 frying chicken (3-4 pounds), skinned and cut into serving pieces
¼ teaspoon white pepper
½ teaspoon Vege-Sal
½ cup artichoke bread stix crumbed
5 tablespoons polyunsaturated oil
3 medium onions, chopped
1 large green pepper, sliced into strips
1 clove garlic, minced
1 cup canned tomatoes
1 cup fresh mushrooms, sliced

Season chicken with pepper and Vege-Sal. Roll in crumbs. Heat oil in skillet and brown chicken on all sides (about 10 minutes). Mix onions, green pepper, garlic, and tomatoes and pour over chicken. Cover. Simmer over low heat 40 minutes. Add mushrooms. Cover and simmer about 15 minutes longer. 4 servings.

TURKEY PLATTER (225 calories)

4 oz. cold sliced turkey
2 slices tomato
2 slices cucumber
lettuce leaves
diet cranberry sauce

Put lettuce on leaves on plate and place turkey on lettuce. Alternate tomato and cucumber slices around turkey. Put small scoop cranberry sauce on one side. 1 serving.

CREAMED CHICKEN WITH MUSHROOMS (190 calories)

3 oz. chicken (white meat) cut up
1 cup skim milk
1 teaspoon polyunsaturated oil
½ cup mushrooms
1/8 teaspoon Vege-Sal
4 slices diet toast

Heat milk and add chicken. Allow to heat through over very low flame (about 10 minutes). Put oil into Teflon pan and saute mushrooms until brown. Add mushrooms to milk/chicken mixture and simmer about 20 minutes. Serve on hot diet toast. 4 servings.

SOUTHERN BAKED CHICKEN (225 calories)
3-pound frying chicken, cut into serving pieces
3 egg whites slightly beaten
1 cup artichoke bread stix crumbs
¼ teaspoon Vege-Sal
¼ cup polyunsaturated oil

Preheat oven to 375 degrees. Mix Vege-Sal with crumbs. Dip chicken into beaten egg whites and then roll in crumbs. Arrange chicken in single layer on shallow baking pan. Pour oil over chicken. Bake uncovered one hour, turning with tongs once or twice to ensure even browning. 6 servings.

VEGETABLES

GRILLED ASPARAGUS (25 calories)
2½ cups cooked asparagus (canned or fresh cooked)
½ cup grated cheese
1½ cups artichoke bread stix crumbed
1 tablespoon polyunsaturated oil
paprika
pepper
    Drain asparagus. Mix cheese, crumbs, and oil together. Add seasonings to taste. Roll asparagus in crumbs. Place on broiler pan. Heat through, turning frequently with tongs to brown evenly. 6 servings.

MARINATED BEETS (40 calories)
1 16-oz. can sliced beets
1 small onion, sliced
1 packet Sweet'n Low or equivalent substitute
3 tablespoons vinegar
¼ teaspoon oregano
    Drain beets, but reserve juice. Place beets and onion in bowl. Combine beet juice, vinegar, sweetener, and oregano. Stir until smooth. Pour over beets and onion and refrigerate until chilled. 4 servings.

STEAMED CARROTS (30 calories)
1 tablespoon polyunsaturated oil
2 cups carrots, sliced
2 tablespoons diced onion
pepper
    Heat oil in Teflon pan. Add remaining ingredients. Cover and steam until vegetables are tender (about 5–8 minutes). 6 servings

STEAMED BROCCOLI (4 oz. = 30 calories)
2 lbs. broccoli
butter (optional)
boiling water
   Cut off and discard large leaves. Wash well. If stems are large, split into pieces. Pierce thick stems in several places with point of sharp knife to encourage even cooking. Cook covered on rack over boiling water 8–15 minutes until broccoli is barely tender. If desired, serve only heads with melted butter as optional dressing. Stems can be reserved for a later meal, to be served cold and slivered as salad or appetizer with vinaigrette dressing. 6–8 servings.

STEAMED BRUSSELS SPROUTS (4 oz. without dressing = 25 calories)
1¼ lbs. Brussels sprouts
½ teaspoon Vege-Sal
butter (optional)
boiling water
   Remove wilted outer leaves. Wash. Cook sprouts seasoned with Vege-Sal, on wired rack over boiling water in covered saucepan. Cook about 10 minutes, or until just tender. Serve plain or with hot melted dressing. 6–8 servings.

CAULIFLOWER (45 calories)
2 packages frozen cauliflower
2 hard-cooked eggs, grated
grated Parmesan cheese
paprika
   Cook cauliflower according to package directions, until barely tender. Drain. Place cauliflower in shallow broiling pan. Sprinkle with eggs, cheese, and paprika. Brown briefly under broiler. 5 servings.

BRAISED CELERY (35 calories)
1 cup celery, cut into ½-inch pieces
2 tablespoons chopped onion
1 tablespoon polyunsaturated oil
2 teaspoons chopped green pepper
½ cup canned tomatoes
½ cup boiling water

152

Put celery in saucepan with boiling water. Simmer 10 minutes. In skillet, heat oil and add onion and green pepper. Saute about 10 minutes over medium heat. Stir in tomatoes and add celery. Simmer 10 minutes longer. 4 servings.

CELERY, PLANTATION STYLE (55 calories)

3 cups celery, cut in 1-inch pieces
1½ cups boiling water
½ teaspoon Vege-Sal
2 tablespoons polyunsaturated oil
2 teaspoons arrowroot
¾ cup skim milk
1 tablespoon finely chopped celery, including leaves
1 tablespoon finely chopped green pepper
1/8 teaspoon onion salt
1/8 teaspoon pepper

Cook celery pieces in boiling water with Vege-Sal until tender (about 10 minutes). Drain and set aside. Heat oil in sauce pan. Blend in arrowroot. Add milk slowly, stirring constantly until sauce thickens. Add remaining ingredients and simmer 2 minutes. Add drained celery. Simmer 5 minutes. Six ½-cup servings.

EGGPLANT PARMIGIANA (170 calories)

1 medium eggplant
2 cups skim milk
2 egg whites, beaten
artichoke bread sticks crumbed
2 oz. mozzarella cheese
tomato sauce (recipe, page 165)

Peel eggplant and cut into ½-inch slices. Soak in cold water overnight. Preheat oven to 350 degrees. Fold milk into beaten egg whites. Dip eggplant into egg-milk batter and roll in crumbs. Place in baking dish and bake 20 minutes or until eggplant is soft. Remove from oven. Place cheese on eggplant and return to oven. Bake until cheese softens. When ready to serve, top with tomato sauce. 4 servings.

GREEN BEANS A LA SPA (25 calories)

⅓ cup polyunsaturated oil
1 clove garlic, sliced thin
1 tablespoon chopped parsley
1 cup canned tomatoes
1 lb. fresh green beans
1 carrot cut into thin strips lengthwise
1 stalk celery, cut into thin strips
1 teaspoon Vege-Sal
1/8 teaspoon pepper

Heat oil in deep skillet. Add garlic and parsley. Saute lightly (about 5 minutes). Add tomatoes and simmer. Wash beans: trim ends. Add beans, carrots, celery to garlic/parsley/tomato mixture. Season. Cover and cook until vegetables are tender (3–6 minutes). 4 servings.

ONIONS OREGANO (60 calories)

12 small white onions
½ teaspoon Vege-Sal
¼ teaspoon white pepper
¾ teaspoon dried oregano
boiling water
½ teaspoon polyunsaturated oil

Peel onions. Barely cover with rapidly boiling water. Add Vege-Sal, pepper, and oil. Simmer 5-6 minutes. Add oregano. Simmer about 5–7 minutes more (according to size of onions) until barely tender but not soft. Drain. 6 servings.

STUFFED PEPPERS (155 calories)

6 green peppers
1 cup ground chuck
1 cup canned tomatoes
1 cup boiled rice (white or brown)
2 tablespoons polyunsaturated oil
1 teaspoon chopped onion
1 teaspoon Vege-Sal
¼ teaspoon pepper
1 cup hot water

Preheat oven to 400 degrees. Wash peppers and cut slice from

154

stem end. Remove seeds and white membrane. Blend other ingredients in bowl. Stuff peppers with mixture and place stuffed peppers in baking dish. Add 1 cup hot water. Bake 30–35 minutes. 6 servings.

CREAMED SPINACH (30 calories)
1 lb. spinach frozen
½ teaspoon Vege-Sal
1 tablespoon polyunsaturated oil
2 teaspoons arrowroot
¾ cup skimmed milk
1/8 teaspoon nutmeg
dash pepper

Cook spinach according to directions, but substitute Vege-Sal for recommended seasoning. Drain and chop fine. Heat oil in saucepan. Add arrowroot, blending well. Slowly blend in milk, stirring constantly until mixture thickens. Add pepper and nutmeg. Add spinach and heat through. 4 servings.

BAKED ACORN SQUASH (50 calories)
2 small acorn squash
½ cup dietetic maple syrup

Preheat oven to 350 degrees. Cut squashes into 4 or more sections each. Remove seeds and stringy pulp. Place in baking pan. Brush cavity and rims of squashes with maple syrup. Cover baking pan with foil and bake until tender (about 20 minutes). 4 servings.

TOMATOES EN CASSEROLE (25 calories)
2 cups stewed tomatoes (canned or fresh)
2 slices onion
3 tablespoons polyunsaturated oil
1 teaspoon Vege-Sal
1/8 teaspoon paprika
1/8 teaspoon pepper

Preheat oven to 350 degrees. Heat oil in skillet. Add onion and seasonings and saute until onion is transparent. Add tomatoes. Mix well. Place in baking dish and bake about 40 minutes, stirring occasionally. 6 servings.

STEWED TOMATOES (30 calories)

1 16-oz. can stewed tomatoes
⅓ cup chopped onion
3 tablespoons chopped green pepper
1 packet Sweet'n Low or equivalent substitute
dash Vege-Sal

Combine ingredients in saucepan. Cover and simmer 10 minutes. 4 servings.

VEGETABLE PANCAKE WITH TOMATO TOPPING (175 calories)

1 pound (total) mixed vegetables, such as:
  asparagus
  broccoli
  carrots
  cauliflower
  onion*
  spinach
  string beans
  (fresh, cooked, leftover, or combination)
½ teaspoon oregano
1 teaspoon Vege-Sal
¼ cup matzo meal
3 egg whites beaten
Water

Place all vegetables in pot in small amount of boiling water or steam over boiling water. Add oregano. Cook until vegetables are barely tender (if raw). Drain. Put vegetables through food grinder. In bowl combine ground up vegetables, Vege-Sal, and matzo meal. Fold in egg whites. Divide into four equal parts and flatten into pancakes. Cook in Teflon pan only long enough to brown, turning once in process.

TOMATO TOPPING

1 15-oz. can salt-free tomatoes
1 package Sweet'n Low or equivalent substitute

Heat tomatoes in pot to full boil. Remove from heat and blend in sweetener. Serve on vegetable pancakes. 4 servings.

*Onion is a must, regardless of other vegetables selected. This is a good way to use leftover vegetables.
If turnip is selected, use only small amount.

156

ZUCCHINI PROVENCALE (25 calories)

2 lbs. zucchini
1 1-lb. can tomatoes
1 small onion, sliced
1 clove garlic, minced

Scrub zucchini well. Trim ends and slice into ¼-inch slices. Cook in small amount of water over low heat until zucchini is almost tender (about five minutes). Drain. Place tomatoes in skillet and mash them into pulp. Add onion and garlic. Simmer 25 minutes. Pour tomato mixture over zucchini and blend. Serve hot. 5 servings.

DESSERTS

APPLESAUCE   (55 calories)

6 tart apples
1¼ packets Sweet'n Low or equivalent substitute
water
optional: lemon juice, cinnamon, nutmeg

Wash, peel, core, and quarter apples. Put in saucepan. Half cover with cold water and bring to boil. Cover. Reduce heat and simmer until apples are tender (8–10 minutes). Stir in sweetener. Cook 5 minutes more. Put apples through sieve. Flavor, if desired, with lemon juice, cinnamon, and/or nutmeg. Serve warm or chilled. 4 servings.

BAKED APPLES   (75 calories)

4 firm apples
1 cup apple juice (unsweetened)
1 packet Sweet'n Low or equivalent substitute
¼ teaspoon cinnamon
¼ teaspoon nutmeg

Preheat oven to 375 degrees. Wash and core apples and put into baking dish, stem side down. Combine juice, sweetener, and spices. Pour over apples. Cover baking dish with foil. Bake approximately 10–12 minutes until soft. 4 servings.

BAKED APRICOT WHIP   (110 calories)

5 egg whites
7 packets Sweet'n Low or equivalent substitute
¼ teaspoon sea salt
¾ teaspoon grated nutmeg
1 cup sieved apricot pulp (water packed or fresh)
2 tablespoons shredded coconut

Preheat oven to 325 degrees. Beat egg whites in bowl until stiff enough to stand in peaks. Blend together sweetener, salt, and nutmeg, and, reserving 1 tablespoonful, fold mixture into egg whites. Fold in apricot pulp. Oil a 2-quart casserole and dust with reserved sweetener mixture. Pour in apricot mixture and top with coconut. Bake until firm in center (about 25 minutes). 8 servings.

BAKED FRESH PEACHES   (55 calories)
4 fresh peaches
apple juice
cinnamon

Preheat oven to 350 degrees. Wash peaches. Dry and place in baking dish. Pour in apple juice to half-fill dish. Sprinkle peaches with cinnamon. Cover dish with foil and bake until peaches are tender (about 20 minutes). 4 servings.

STEWED FRUIT IN SYRUP   (7 calories)
2 cups any preferred fruit (apricots, peaches, pears, plums)
4 packets Sweet'n Low or equivalent substitute
1 tablespoon lemon juice

Boil sweetener and lemon juice and add fruit. Simmer until softened (8–10 minutes).

JELLO CAKE   (35 calories)
1 package diet Jello (any flavor)
6 thin graham crackers
½ cup nondairy whip topping

Prepare Jello according to directions on package. Pour in shallow pan and chill until firm. Whip nondairy topping until stiff. Put a graham cracker on each of 6 small dessert plates. Cut jello into 6 squares and top crackers with jello. Put 1 tablespoon topping on each mound of jello. 6 servings.

LEMON-PINEAPPLE JELLO WHIP   (35 calories)
1 package diet lemon Jello
2 cups boiling water
2 cups unsweetened pineapple juice
¼–½ cup nondairy topping

Combine jello and hot water. Stir until jello dissolves. Add pineapple juice and refrigerate until very firm. In chilled bowl, whip topping until stiff. Using slow speed on mixer, blend in firm jello.. Eight 3-oz. servings.

159

CHOCOLATE MOUSSE (60 calories)
1 package Chocolate Diet Pudding
1 cup nondairy topping (Whirlwhip)
1 egg white

Follow package directions to make chocolate pudding. Cool. In chilled bowl of electric mixer, combine topping and egg white. Beat until stiff. Blend in pudding, using slowest speed of mixer. Twelve 3-oz. servings.

COFFEE MOUSSE (35 calories)
1 package Vanilla Diet Pudding
2 teaspoons instant coffee
1 cup nondairy topping
1 egg white

Follow package directions to make pudding, adding instant coffee to basic pudding mixture. Complete recipe by following directions given above for Chocolate Mousse. Twelve 3-oz. servings.

COCONUT MOUSSE (35 calories)
1 package Vanilla Diet Pudding
4 drops coconut extract
¼ cup shredded coconut (toasted)
1 cup nondairy topping
1 egg white

Follow package directions to make pudding, adding coconut extract for flavoring. Toast coconut under broiler and sprinkle over pudding before chilling. Complete recipe by following directions given above for Chocolate Mousse. Twelve 3-oz. servings.

PEAR COMPOTE (55 calories)
4 fresh pears
3 cups syrup for stewed fruits (recipe, page 159)

Wash and peel pears. Simmer in syrup until tender (8–10 minutes). Chill. 4 servings.

PINEAPPLE ICE CREAM   (35 calories)
¼ medium pineapple, very ripe
4 oz. evaporated skim milk, frozen
2 packets Sweet'n Low or equivalent substitute

Strip pineapple of its outside rind. Chop pineapple into small pieces. Place in blender and blend for a few seconds. (You can use the entire pineapple, if you wish, and make four times the recipe or reserve ¾ of pineapple for other uses.) Place pineapple to be used for ice cream in foil and store in freezer. When ready to make ice cream, remove frozen pineapple and milk from freezer and let stand at room temperature 10 minutes. Chop milk and fruit. Place in chilled stainless steel bowl of your mixer and mix at low speed until smooth. Add sweetener. Raise speed to high. Beat until mixture doubles in volume. Serve immediately or store in refrigerator until serving time. Upon serving, the mixture should have the consistency of "store-bought" ice cream. 6 servings.

STEWED PRUNES   (100 calories)
1 lb. dried prunes
water
dash lemon juice

Wash prunes. Soak in cold water 12 hours. Heat prunes slowly in water in which they've been soaking. When water simmers, lower flame. Cover and simmer until skins are tender and water has reduced and thickened. Add lemon juice during cooking period. 8 servings.

STRAWBERRY BAVARIAN   (35 calories)
1 envelope Knox unflavored gelatin
¼ cup cold water
¾ cup boiling water
6 packets Sweet'n Low or equivalent substitute
1 teaspoon lemon juice
12 whole frozen strawberries
2 oz. evaporated skimmed milk, frozen in ice tray

Soften gelatin in cold water. Add boiling water and stir until dissolved. Let stand for a few minutes. Put strawberries and frozen milk into blender. Add gelatin mixture. Blend until smooth and pour into individual sherbet glasses or larger glass bowl. Refrigerate. 4 servings.

SANDWICHES

OPEN-FACE GRILLED CHEESE SANDWICH (160 calories)
4 slices diet bread toasted
4 slices low-fat hard cheese (skim-milk)
4 slices tomato

Place toast on sheet pan and top with cheese. Broil long enough for cheese to melt. Serve with tomato slice. 4 servings.

OPEN-FACE TURKEY SANDWICH (175 calories)
4 slices diet bread
4 slices turkey (white)
4 slices tomato
4 small lettuce leaves

Place lettuce on bread, then turkey, then tomato. 4 servings.

TUNA SANDWICH (200 calories)
One 7-oz. can water-packed tuna, drained and flaked.
½ cup diced celery
1 tablespoon minced onion
1 teaspoon lemon juice
1 tablespoon Balanaise mayonnaise
¼ teaspoon Vege-Sal
4 slices diet bread

Blend first six ingredients in bowl. Divide between the four slices of bread. 4 servings.

SAUCES, DRESSINGS AND MARINADES

COCKTAIL SAUCE   (18 calories)
6 tablespoons salt-free catsup
2 tablespoons horseradish (bottled)
4 tablespoons lemon juice
dash celery salt
dash Tabasco Sauce
    Combine first 4 ingredients in blender. Blend thoroughly. Add Tabasco to taste. Serve with seafood.

HERB SAUCE   (30 calories)
1 shallot, minced
½ teaspoon minced celery
½ teaspoon minced fennel
½ teaspoon minced fresh parsley
½ teaspoon fresh sweet marjoram, minced, or ¼ teaspoon powdered
    marjoram
¼ teaspoon powdered sage or ½ teaspoon minced fresh sage
2 tablespoons butter
white wine or cider vinegar
2 tablespoons olive oil
    Melt butter in small saucepan over medium heat. Add shallot and saute gently 3 minutes. Add all other herbs and seasonings. Barely cover with preferred vinegar (wine or cider). Simmer 10 minutes. Blend in olive oil. Yield: 1 cup (approximately). Serve hot over boiled beef, grilled or baked fish, chicken, and veal.

"INSTANT" HOLLANDAISE SAUCE   (40 calories)
½ cup Balanaise mayonnaise
2 tablespoons hot water
1 teaspoon lemon juice
    Put mayonnaise in top of double boiler over hot water. Blend 2 tablespoons hot water into mayonnaise. Heat through. Remove from heat and blend in lemon juice. Serve with asparagus or other vegetables or over poached eggs. Yield: ½ cup.

163

LEMON PARSLEY SAUCE (25 calories)
¼ cup chopped parsley
1 small onion, diced
¼ cup lemon juice
    Combine all ingredients. Serve with any fish.

LEMON SAUCE (40 calories)
1 packet Sweet'n Low or equivalent substitute
1 tablespoon arrowroot
¼ teaspoon Vege-Sal
1 cup boiling water
1 teaspoon polyunsaturated oil
grated rind of ½ lemon
1 tablespoon lemon juice
    Combine sweetener, arrowroot, and Vege-Sal and mix
thoroughly. Slowly add boiling water and stir until mixture thickens.
Gradually add oil. Stir until mixture is smooth. Add grated lemon
rind and juice and blend well. 4–5 servings with broiled filet of sole
or other broiled fish.

MINT SAUCE (35 calories)
2 tablespoons dry mint or 4 tablespoons fresh chopped mint
2 packets Sweet'n Low or equivalent substitute
½ cup apple cider vinegar
    Place mint in bowl. Add sweetener and vinegar. Blend. Let
stand 1 hour or more before serving.

TERIYAKI STEAK SAUCE (50 calories)
1 cup soy sauce
4 cloves garlic, crushed
2 packets Sweet'n Low or equivalent substitute
2 tablespoons lemon juice
2 tablespoons Worcestershire Sauce
2 tablespoons polyunsaturated oil
pepper to taste
    Mix all ingredients together. Marinate steak in sauce 5–6 hours
or longer, turning periodically. Pierce steak with fork to allow sauce
to penetrate meat.

TOMATO SAUCE (½ cup, 40 calories)

1 15-oz. can salt-free tomatoes

1 small onion, diced

1 teaspoon oregano

1 stalk celery, diced

Blend ingredients in medium-sized pot. Simmer over low heat 1 hour.

SPECIAL CAESAR SALAD DRESSING (65 calories)

1 teaspoon Dijon mustard

½ teaspoon Sweet'n Low or equivalent substitute

1 teaspoon lemon juice

2 tablespoons tarragon vinegar

2 tablespoons olive oil

2 tablespoons safflower oil

1 egg

1 garlic clove minced or ½ teaspoon garlic powder

2 artichoke bread stix crushed to crumbs

Mix all ingredients together, including egg, using low speed on blender. Use with mixture of iceberg and romaine lettuce. Instead of traditional croutons, sprinkle salad with artichoke bread stix crumbs after tossing with dressing.

FRENCH DRESSING (60 calories per tablespoon)

One 14-oz. bottle salt-free catsup

1½ cups safflower oil

¼ teaspoon dry mustard

1 teaspoon Vege-Sal

1 teaspoon paprika

1 tablespoon Sweet'n Low or equivalent substitute

1 egg

Mix dry ingredients. Add catsup and egg and mix well. Put into blender. With blender at lowest speed, add oil gradually. When well mixed, increase blender speed for a few moments. Yield: about 1½ pints. Store in refrigerator in covered jar or bowl.

VINAIGRETTE DRESSING   (8 calories per tablespoon)
⅔ cup white vinegar
⅓ cup water
½ cup chopped green pepper, scallions, and pimento
Sweet'n Low to taste, or equivalent substitute

Mix ingredients. Let stand 5 or more hours before serving. Yield: 1½ cups.

MARINADE   (328 calories, total recipe)
3 tablespoons safflower oil
3 tablespoons vinegar
3 tablespoons lemon juice
½ teaspoon Vege-Sal
½ teaspoon pepper

Combine all ingredients. Shake in bottle to blend well, or blend with mixer, using lowest speed. Chill before using.

HERBS AND SPICES
(Good Partners For Sodium-Restricted Diets)

When your physican tells you to restrict your salt intake, don't believe you've been condemned to a lifetime of dull, bland food. With the exercise of just a little imagination, you can eat tastier, more interesting food than ever before.

Under various headings below are listed herbs and spices to add flavor sparkle to basic foods—from scrambled eggs to meat, fish, and poultry dishes; soups; vegetables; desserts and sauces too. Choose any one of the herbs or spices listed as good partners, or experiment and combine two or three from the appropriate list. Always use a gentle wrist, remembering that the mark of the good cook is a subtle blending of flavors—that less is generally better than more.

Even if you are an apartment dweller, you can have your own herb garden. A window-box garden can provide those special items that you may not readily find in your supermarket or vegetable stand, and if you should be fortunate enough to buy a hydroponic garden, you can grow indoors, even in wildest weather, not only herbs but a great variety of vegetables, including tomatoes. And don't overlook what flowers can contribute to your meals in terms of taste and talk, as, for instance, rose petals in a fruit drink or dessert, or even in certain soups; and, in salad, nasturtium leaves or minced marigold petals—but use sparingly! Please don't, however, experiment on your own with flowers. Some of the prettiest are poisonous. But the list of herbs and spices below should provide you with plenty of room for experimentation and new taste pleasures.

APPETIZERS
Cottage cheese in celery sticks—sprinkle with sesame seed.
Tomato juice—sprinkle with a dash of mace or tarragon.
Vegetable juice—dust with crushed dried thyme or oregano.
Raw cauliflower—serve with dip of diet yogurt blended with lemon, paprika, and mustard, or with a dash of horseradish.

167

Cherry tomatoes—serve with dressing of olive oil, lemon juice, minced parsley, and minced garlic.

Fruit cup—place 1 fresh rosemary leaf in each cup 10 minutes before serving, or garnish each cup with ¼ teaspoon chopped fresh rose petal, or garnish cup with 1 tiny rose petal.

EGGS

Chervil, chives, cumin, curry, mustard (ground), fresh minced mustard leaves, onion, onion powder, paprika, parsley, pepper, sage, savory, scallions, shallots, tarragon, thyme, watercress.

FISH AND SHELLFISH

Bay leaf, cayenne pepper, celery salt, chives, curry, dill, fennel seed, garlic, marjoram, oregano, paprika, parsley, pepper, savory, scallions, shallots, tarragon, thyme, watercress.

MEAT

Allspice, anise seed, bay leaf, caraway seed, cayenne pepper, celery salt, chili powder, cloves, cumin seed, dill, garlic, ginger, lemon, onion, oregano, paprika, parsley, pepper, rosemary, sage, scallions, sesame seed, tarragon, thyme, watercress.

POULTRY

Anise, sweet basil, bay leaf, chives, cumin, garlic powder, ginger, lemon, marjoram, oregano, rosemary, saffron, sage, savory, scallions, sesame seed, shallots, tarragon, thyme.

SALADS AND SALAD DRESSINGS

Bay leaf, caraway seed, celery seed, chervil, chili, dill, fennel, garlic, lemon, marigold, nasturtium, onion, onion flakes, paprika, parsley, poppy seed, scallions, sesame seed, tarragon, thyme, watercress.

SOUPS

Allspice (green pea soup), basil, bayleaf, celery, chervil, chives, cinnamon, curry, garlic, mace, mint, onion, oregano, paprika, parsley, scallions, shallots, sorrel, watercress.

VEGETABLES

Allspice (with cabbage, carrots, tomatoes), anise, sweet basil, bay leaf, cinnamon, cumin, dill, fennel, garlic, ginger (particularly with spinach), mace, marjoram, nutmeg (particularly with spinach), onion powder, oregano, poppy seed, sage, scallions, shallots, tarragon, thyme.

"AUX FINES HERBES," FRESH

1 teaspoon chopped chervil
1 teaspoon chopped chives
2 tablespoons chopped parsley
1 teaspoon chopped tarragon or ½ teaspoon dried tarragon

Select fresh young leaves. Wash thoroughly. Dry. Mince fine. Use as garnish for 4 servings fish, roast, steak, or cook in soup or stew.

FRESH BOUQUET GARNI

1 sprig parsley
1 sprig savory
1 sprig chervil
2 stalks celery, including leaves
1 small sprig basil
6 leaves chives

Select young fresh herbs. Wash thoroughly and tie in bundle with white thread. At beginning of cooking period, place in liquid for meat stews or meat or vegetable soups.

Chapter 14

Low-Calorie Holiday Cookbook

THE Harbor Island weight-control philosophy encourages you to forget your diet one day a week, and a holiday is certainly a good time to take advantage of that dietary freedom. But, while it's expected you'll exceed your usual caloric allowance, even on a holiday there is no point in eating beyond satiety.

This holiday cookbook incorporates traditional foods and traditional bounty, but with low-calorie ingredients wherever feasible and Harbor Island's own low-calorie variations. Sometimes there are low-calorie alternatives for holiday desserts—Pesach Apple Fluff, for instance, instead of traditional apple pie for supper at the conclusion of Yom Kippur and Pumpkin Custard a la Spa for the traditional pumpkin pie of Thanksgiving—and for standbys like crumbled artichoke breadsticks substituting for traditional bread stuffings for turkey and chicken.

If, in the desserts, you miss certain traditions, as where the Harbor Island Spa's Cranberry Mold is substituted for traditional plum pudding or mince pie at Christmas, remember that no food was a tradition when first eaten. In this holiday cookbook from Harbor Island Spa, we hope you'll find recipes you enjoy so much they'll become traditional with you.

Since the holiday meals are generous, it's suggested that breakfast be restricted to low-calorie juice or half a grapefruit, plus one soft-boiled egg or small serving of cottage cheese, and that other meals of the day be restricted to calorie-free or low-calorie vegetables and snacks and a low-calorie form of a modest amount of complete protein, such as one slice of white meat of turkey or a small slice of fish. The only breakfast menus contained in the cookbook are listed for Passover. When the holiday lasts several days, such as

Chanukah, it is expected that you will restrict your caloric count while continuing to include traditional foods. We think you'll be astonished at how delicious some of the Spa's low-calorie versions are—Harbor Island Spa Cheese Cake, for instance, or Easter Sparkle dessert, which contains no calories at all but contributes a shimmering yellow-green climax for this spring celebration.

THANKSGIVING

Thanksgiving celebration without turkey and pumpkin would be unthinkable, and most of us serve them believing them to be the discoveries of the Pilgrims from the Indians. In truth, the Pilgrims knew and enjoyed turkey in England, the bird having first been taken to Spain from Mexico by 16th-century Spanish voyagers. Most of us serve pumpkin pie thinking this delicacy too was a favorite of the early Americans, quite forgetting that spices did not rate high priority at that time when survival was first order of the day. Actually pumpkin pie—any kind of dessert pie—did not come into being in America until the early 19th century, so it is possible that the earliest form of enjoyment of pumpkin as dessert was a variation on Harbor Island Spa's own Pumpkin Custard. Pumpkin itself was known in England and Europe 50 years after Columbus discovered America. It was then called "Turkish cucumber" because, somehow, its usage in Europe spread through Turkey. America's Indians called the versatile vegetable "pompion." The pilgrims stewed pompion with Indian (corn) meal and made bread from it—as well as serving pompion as a vegetable.

MENU	CALORIES PER SERVING
Celery sticks, raw zucchini slivers, radishes	0
4 oz. roast turkey with artichoke (stix) stuffing	225
2 oz. cranberry sauce	25
½ cup mashed white potatoes	50
1 tablespoon giblet gravy	50
¼ acorn squash, baked	50
4 oz. broccoli, steamed	30
3 oz. Pumpkin Custard a la Spa	61
	———
	491

CHRISTMAS

Our Christmas traditions come primarily from England insofar as food is concerned but most Americans substitute turkey for the more traditional goose. The menu below, however, calls for goose, but the traditional plum pudding gives way to a glamorous, delicious, low-calorie substitute: Cranberry Mold.

MENU	CALORIES PER SERVING
Relish boat: carrot slivers, radishes, celery slices	0
4 oz. roast goose with apple/orange stuffing	348
½ cup applesauce	55
½ cup pickled beets	55
½ cup steamed carrots	30
1 Cup of Gold, Flambe	158
3 oz. Cranberry Mold	40
	686

NEW YEAR'S DAY

The primary culinary tradition for New Year's Day is roast beef, and that's included in the menu below. The low calorie recommendation is Chocolate Mousse as dessert.

MENU	CALORIES PER SERVING
Raw vegetable relish plate: cherry tomatoes, radishes, celery sticks	0
4 oz. prime ribs of beef	300
½ cup mashed potato	50
½ cup steamed carrots	30
½ cup steamed Brussels sprouts	25
3 oz. Chocolate Mousse	35
	440

EASTER

Since ham and leg of lamb are equally traditional Easter fare, our menu specifies lamb prepared with simplicity to put the focus on the fresh taste of spring lamb. The pretty sparkling dessert is as delicious as it's pretty and contains no calories at all.

MENU	CALORIES PER SERVING
4 oz. roast leg of lamb with mint sauce	325
1 roasted white potato	80
½ cup steamed baby carrots	30
2 oz. asparagus vinaigrette	20
1 cup Spring salad	25
3 oz. Easter Sparkle	0
	480

PASSOVER

Except for Passover, no breakfast (or lunch or supper) menus are included. In general, we recommend that you reduce your calories at these meals to a minimum but, at breakfast at least, you obtain some form of animal protein—1 soft-boiled egg, or ½ cup of low-calorie cottage cheese, or 2 ounces turkey, or 2 ounces of lox.

Passover marks the flight of the Jews from bondage in Egypt after the death of Joseph. The eating of matzos is a tradition, the substitute for bread invented by the Jews when, escaping from Egypt, they could spend no time preparing food. Flour and water, without leavening, was rolled thin on flat boards and carried by the escaping Jews to bake under the hot sun.

The first two nights of Passover are traditionally spent in family gatherings known as the "Seder," wherein the story of the Exodus is retold with food, ritual, and song. The tablecloth, as on other holidays, is white, and only the best china and silver is used. Each place is set with a wine goblet, with wine to be drunk at intervals during the service. Since the calorie count will vary according to the type of wine you use, no calories for wine are listed in the menus below.

A traditional seder platter is placed at the head of the table. On it are symbolic items—hard-cooked eggs, charoses (a mixture of apples, nuts, and honey), bitter herbs (horseradish), radishes, a lamb shank bone, a dish of salt water, parsley to be dipped into the water, and the Kiddish cup or goblet.

During the services, the "Feer Kashas"—the four questions concerning the reasons for the various traditions, such as the eating of the matzos—are asked by the youngest male present and answered by the father or rabbi.

PASSOVER BREAKFAST MENUS

BREAKFAST #1	CALORIES PER SERVING
4 oz. fresh orange juice	90
1 matzo brie	200
1 tablespoon fruit preserve	50
Coffee, tea, Sanka, nonfat milk	1-3
	241-243

BREAKFAST #2	
½ grapefruit	50
Egg in mushroom cup	110
1 toasted matzo	100
Coffee, tea, Sanka, nonfat milk	1-3
	261-263

BREAKFAST #3	
4 oz. stewed figs	75
4 oz. creamed finnan haddie on toasted matzo	356
Beverage	1-3
	432-434

BREAKFAST #4	
½ cantaloupe	50
4 oz. salted mackerel	345
1 toasted matzo	100
Beverage	1-3
	496-498

174

BREAKFAST #5

3 oz. stewed prunes	75
3-egg omelette with 1 tablespoon strawberry preserve	295
1 matzo	100
Beverage	1-3
	471-473

PASSOVER DINNERS

FIRST SEDER

On Table: First and Second Seder: Sprig parsley
1 lamb shank bone
Bitter herbs
Charoses
Salt water
Hard-cooked egg

MENU	*CALORIES PER SERVING*
3 oz. gefilte fish with horseradish	150
1 cup chicken broth with matzo ball	175
4 oz. brisket of beef	450
4 oz. carrot/sweet potato tzimmes	65
4 oz. asparagus vinaigrette	20
1 maccaroon	15
	875

SECOND SEDER

MENU	*CALORIES PER SERVING*
3 oz. gefilte fish with horseradish	150
1 cup schav, garnished with parsley and pareve knaidlach	130
4 oz. roast chicken with artichoke (stix) stuffing	250
½ cup green beans almondine	25
1 matzo	100
Matzo meal sponge cake	140
	795

175

ROSH HASHANAH

Celebrating this holiday ushering in the New Year, the time of new hope, it is traditional to feature one or more "sweet" dishes on the holiday table. As a sweet item is placed on the table, it is traditional for Bubeh (Grandmother) to say, "For a sweet year." In the menu below, the sweet items are prune and sweet potato tzimmes, but served without the brisket of beef with which the tzimmes are prepared, and taiglach, a cakelike dessert with honey, citron, and nuts. (The brisket and leftover tzimmes are held over for delicious reheating next day.)

MENU	CALORIES PER SERVING
3 oz. gefilte fish garnished with horseradish with beets	150
1 cup chicken broth with farfel	55
4 oz. roast chicken or capon with artichoke (stix) stuffing	320
½ cup prune and sweet potato tzimmes (without brisket)	125
Tossed lettuce, tomato, radish, cucumber salad	25
1 taiglach	210
	885

YOM KIPPUR

This holiday, most solemn of the Jewish year, is marked by a day of fasting when Jews atone for past sins and ask the Lord for forgiveness. During the 24-hour fasting period, from sundown of the evening before Yom Kippur, no food or water may pass the lips, so that food before this holiday is simple and free of anything highly seasoned or salted. Even after the fasting period, food tends to be lighter than the norm for festive Jewish fare.

MENU FOR EREV-YOM KIPPUR	CALORIES PER SERVING

(Food served just before sundown and the start of the Yom Kippur observance.)

2″ wedge honeydew melon	50
1 cup schav, garnished with parsley	55
4 oz. brisket with prune and sweet potato tzimmes	390
4 oz. potato kugel	115

176

4 oz. peas and carrots	55
2 oz. cranberry sauce	25
3 oz. orange gelatin salad with carrots	25
\Apple rings \	60
	———
	775

For the end of the period of fasting, here is a Harbor Island Spa

MENU	*CALORIES PER SERVING*
½ cup cantaloupe balls	25
4-oz. cup cold beet borsch	65
4 oz. broiled whitefish	210
½ cup mixed carrots, peas, turnips	75
Pesach apple fluff \	40
	———
	415

SHAVUOTH

Shavuoth, or Feast of Weeks, commemorating the giving of the Torah by God to Moses, falls precisely seven weeks after the second day of Passover. This holiday, a joyous celebration of the harvest, originally called for every farmer to place the first fruit of the harvest in a gold, silver, or wicker basket and take it to the Temple as a thank-offering to the Lord for his bounty.

It is customary to decorate the home with plants and flowers as reminder of the green mountains of Sinai and to read aloud the story of Ruth and her acceptance of the Jewish faith. On Shavuoth Eve, after the traditional candles are lighted in the home, it is custom to go to the synagogue to worship. It is custom too that, in commemorating the giving of the Ten Commandments to Moses, boys and girls who have studied Hebrew are confirmed on Shavuoth morning.

Meals during this holiday feature dairy foods.

MENU	*CALORIES PER SERVING*
3 oz. gefilte fish with beet horseradish	150
½ cup cream of tomato soup	40
2 cheese blintzes (recipes for traditional and low-calorie)	175*
½ cup marinated cucumbers	18

2″ wedge, Harbor Island Spa Cheese Cake   67
Fruit bowl (optional)

                                                                450

*350 calories for traditional version

SUKKOTH

A joyful holiday lasting a week, Sukkoth marks the gathering of the harvest. Fruits and vegetables are features at Sukkoth meals. Among the favorites are holeskes (stuffed cabbage) and strudel, that most delicious of all Jewish pastries.

MENU	CALORIES PER SERVING
1 small apple sliced, sprinkled with cinnamon and lemon juice	70
6 oz. holeskes	140
4 oz. carrot and fresh pineapple mold	40
1 average serving mixed fruit strudel	225
	475

CHANUKAH

This joyous holiday, lasting eight days, traditionally features potato pancakes and potato kugel (pudding). Commemorating the victory of the Maccabees over Antiochus of Syria and the rededication of the defiled Temple of Jerusalem, Chanukah is marked by the lighting of another candle in the Menorah each night for eight nights until eight candles are alight. Traditionally, each night of Chanukah, when the candle or candles are lit, presents are distributed among the family, celebrating the right of Jews to worship the Lord in their Temple.
MENU
A variety of holiday foods, but, inevitably, Chanukah potato latkes (pancakes) and potato kugel.

PURIM

Joyous is the word for Purim (the Feast of Esther), honoring the beautiful Queen of a non-Jewish King who triumphed over the wicked Haman who tried to undermine the Jews in the mind of the King.

Traditional delicacy at Purim are hamantaschen, a pastry filled with poppy seeds and honey and walnuts, and shaped into a tiny tricorn "hat," reminder of the ones Haman wore.

Calories watchers should choose the tiniest possible "hat," and never more than one.

MENU	CALORIES PER SERVING
½ chopped egg with onion	43
4 oz. beet borsch with 1 teaspoon sour cream	65
4 oz. stuffed breast of veal with artichoke (stix) stuffing	335
½ cup leaf spinach	30
¼ acorn squash	50
1 dill pickle	10
One 2" hamantaschen	240
	773

HOLIDAY SOUPS AND SOUP ACCOMPANIMENTS

BORSCH

1 lb. lean beef, cubed
1 soup bone
1 chicken (3–4 pounds), cut-up
3 carrots, chopped
3 small onions, sliced
3 stalks celery, including tops, diced
3 quarts water
¼ teaspoon whole peppercorns
½ bay leaf
1 spray thyme
2 laurel leaves (optional)
1 sprig parsley
salt and pepper
2 beets, pared and chopped
sour cream for garnish

Put beef, bone, chicken, carrots, onions, celery, and water in large pot. Bring slowly to boil. Tie spices and herbs in small cloth bag and put in pot. Add parsley. simmer, covered, approximately 2 hours. Strain. Set meat aside for other use. Season broth to taste. Add beets and cook 15 minutes. Strain. Reheat. Serve with topping of sour cream. To serve cold, refrigerate a minimum of 2 hours. Approximate yield: 2 quarts. One-half-cup serving, 65 calories.

SCHAV

2 lbs. schav (sorrel, sour grass)
1 onion, grated
3 quarts water
1 teaspoon salt
2 tablespoons lemon juice
4 envelopes Sweet'n Low or equivalent substitute
2 eggs
sour cream as garnish

Wash schav 2 or 3 times in cold water and then wash in lukewarm water. Combine schav, onion, water, salt in large pot. Bring to boil. Lower heat and cook over low heat 1 hour. Mix lemon juice and sweetener and add to schav mixture. Cook 15 minutes. Taste, and adjust seasonings if necessary. Remove schav from stove. Beat eggs in large bowl and add slowly to schav, stirring constantly to prevent curdling. Refrigerate until serving time. Serve with sour cream garnish. 8 servings. One-cup serving with 1 teaspoon sour cream equals 55 calories.

FARFEL

1½ cups flour
½ teaspoon salt
2 eggs, beaten

Sift flour and salt. Place on board, make a well of flour and drop in one egg. Work into flour. Drop in second egg. Work flour/eggs until dough is formed. Roll a piece of this stiff dough into a long, thin, round strip. Form all the dough into similar long, thin strips. Let dry at room temperature until strip can be chopped into tiny pieces about the size of small peas. Continue drying process. Finally put farfel on tray and bake in 325-degree oven for 15 minutes or until completely dry. As a soup accompaniment, 2 tablespoons equal approximately 18 calories.

MANDLEN (PASSOVER)

3 egg yolks, beaten
¾ cup matzo cake meal
1 teaspoon salt
pepper, dash
3 tablespoons potato flour
3 egg whites, stiffly beaten
polyunsaturated oil for deep frying

Beat cake meal into beaten egg yolks. Add seasonings and blend. Gradually add potato flour. Fold in egg whites and blend thoroughly. Heat fat in deep fryer (French fryer is helpful). Drop batter into hot fat by teaspoonful. Fry until well browned. Remove balls with slotted spoon and drain on paper towels. Crisp in hot oven before using as garnish in chicken broth or other favorite soup. 8-10 servings. Approximately 83 calories per serving.

PAREVE KNAIDLACH

2 egg yolks
½ teaspoon salt
2 egg whites, stiffly beaten
½ cup matzo meal

Beat the egg yolks and salt until thick. Fold into the egg whites. Now gradually fold in the matzo meal. Chill one hour. Moisten hands. Shape mixture into ½-inch balls. Cook in boiling salted water 20 minutes. Serve in dairy or meat soups. Makes about 16 balls. Two balls equal approximately 75 calories.

CHEESE DISHES

CHEESE BLINTZES

6 eggs, beaten
1 tablespoon potato flour
½ cup water
1 lb. farmer cheese (pot cheese)
½ lb. diet cottage cheese (drained of any liquid)
2 egg yolks
½ teaspoon cinnamon
¼ cup seedless yellow raisins
2 envelopes Sweet'n Low or equivalent substitute
2-3 tablespoons polyunsaturated oil (unless you use Teflon pan)

Combine flour and water. Add the six beaten eggs and beat together well. Place a little oil on medium-size skillet, or use crepe pan. Heat over medium heat. When hot, drop in one small ladle of batter, turning pan so that batter spreads all over skillet. When brown on bottom side, turn out on towel (paper or, preferably, a tea towel) with browned side up.

Combine the two cheeses. Add egg yolks, cinnamon, raisins, and sweetener. Place 2 tablespoons of cheese mixture on each round pancake. Fold in ends and then roll up pancake. Heat remaining tablespoon of oil in skillet. Place blintzes in skillet, turning twice to make sure the blintzes are browned on all sides. Remove to platter. Serve with sour cream or applesauce. Six servings. Two blintzes approximately 350 calories.

LOW-CALORIE CHEESE BLINTZES

1 pound diet cottage cheese
4 eggs
2 tablespoons presifted (or Wondra) flour

Put ingredients in blender and spin until well blended. Use Teflon to avoid use of oil on griddle. Dip or pour mixture into 3–4 "pancakes" and brown nicely on one side and then other. Roll up. There is no extra filling for these "blintzes."

Serve with low-calorie maple syrup or low-calorie jelly or 1 teaspoon honey. Not counting sweet accompaniment, each blintz is about 86 calories. 3–4 servings.

EGG DISHES

EGGS AND ONIONS
8 hard-cooked eggs
¾ cup chopped onions
¼ teaspoon Vege-Sal
¼ teaspoon pepper
3 tablespoons rendered chicken fat

Chop the eggs and onions together until very fine. Blend in the Vege-Sal, pepper, and fat. Chill. Arrange on lettuce leaves. 6–10 servings as appetizer. 2-ounce serving, 43 calories.

EGGS IN MUSHROOM CUPS
6 large mushrooms
polyunsaturated oil
¾ teaspoon Vege-Sal
6 eggs
parsley, chopped fine, as garnish

Choose large "cup shaped" mushrooms. Wipe with damp paper towel. Remove stalk very close to the cup so as to leave slight hollow and season mushrooms with part of Vege-Sal. Heat mushroom caps with part of oil in skillet. When mushrooms are partially cooked, remove from the pan and carefully break an egg into each mushroom cup. Dust the eggs with Vege-Sal. Add additional oil to skillet and return mushrooms to skillet. Baste the eggs with the oil, spooning it over the eggs until the eggs are set to desired degree of firmness. Carefully remove the eggs in their mushroom cups from the hot oil, using a perforated fish slice so that the excess oil will drip away. Transfer to heated platter or to hot individual serving dishes. Sprinkle with chopped parsley and serve immediately. Each egg in mushroom equals approximately 110 calories.

MATZO BREI
(Fried Matzos and Eggs)
4 eggs
1 teaspoon grated onion or
1 onion, diced or sliced (optional)
4 matzos
¼ teaspoon Vege-Sal
¼ teaspoon pepper
1 tablespoon polyunsaturated oil

Beat eggs and mix in grated onion (if used) and seasoning. Heat fat in skillet. If diced or sliced onion used, saute onions in hot fat until transparent. Meantime, place matzos in bowl of cold water for several minutes. Squeeze and drain matzos and crumble into egg mixture. Turn mixture into pan. Heat over low flame until browned, then turn to other side. Serve garnished with strawberry jam. 4 servings. 186 calories per serving.

FISH DISHES

BOILED CARP

2 lbs. carp (or other fish)
½ medium onion
2 tablespoons celery, diced
1 carrot, diced
½ teaspoon mixed who spices
3 cups water
2 tablespoons white vinegar
½ teaspoon Vege-Sal
¼ teaspoon pepper
parsley garnish

Cut fish into four portions. Put other ingredients into pot and bring to boil. When water boils, reduce heat to low flame. Add fish and cook until flesh leaves the bones (about 20 minutes). Carefully remove bones. Put fish on heated platter. Garnish with parsley. 4 servings. 100 calories per 4-oz. serving. As appetizer, 8 servings.

Strain broth and reserve in refrigerator for future use. When jellied, it can be cut into cubes and served with cold fish, or it can be used hot as base for fish soup or fish chowder.

CREAMED FINNAN HADDIE

3 lbs. finnan haddie or smoked cod
2 quarts water
3 tablespoons butter
3 tablespoons flour
1 cup skim milk
2 egg yolks, beaten
½ teaspoon Vege-Sal
pepper, dash

Soak fish overnight in cold water. Remove fish and discard water. Wash fish in running cold water, then dry with paper towels.

Cut fish into 3- or 4-inch pieces. Put with water in large pot over medium flame. After water comes to boil, cook 5 minutes. Remove fish, and flake. Melt butter in small saucepan. Add flour, blending well, and cook, stirring constantly, 1 minute. Add milk gradually, stirring constantly. Mix tablespoon of hot liquid into egg yolks. Blend. Add egg yolks to cream sauce. stirring constantly. Add seasonings and flaked fish. Serve hot on slice of toasted diet bread. 4-oz. serving equals 356 calories.

FRIED SALT MACKEREL

2 lbs. salt mackerel
3 tablespoons flour
¼ teaspoon Vege-Sal
pepper, dash
3 tablespoons polyunsaturated oil
1 large onion, sliced

Soak mackerel overnight in cold water. Clean fish thoroughly, removing head and tail. Roll fish in flour seasoned with Vege-Sal and pepper. Heat oil in frying pan. When hot, put in fish. Fry until brown on one side, then turn and fry on other side. While fish is cooking, add onions to oil/fish. Cook onions, stirring occasionally, until golden. Remove fish and onions to heated serving platter. 4-6 servings. 3 oz. equal 205 calories.

Optional garnish: pickled pears with cinnamon or cloves.

PICKLED HERRING

6 fillets of miltz herring
4 onions, sliced thin
1 cup white vinegar
¼ cup water
2 packages Sweet'n Low or equivalent substitute
2 teaspoons pickling spice
2 bay leaves

Wash herring thoroughly and soak in cold water for 6 hours. Drain. Cut the herring into 2-inch pieces. In a bowl or glass jar, alternate layers of herring and onions. Bring vinegar, water, sweetener, pickling spice, and bay leaves to boil. Remove from heat. Cool slightly and pour over herring. Cover tightly. Shake. Refrigerate for 48 hours before serving.

For dairy meals, the liquid may be mixed with sour cream (2 tablespoons) before or after pickling.

The herring may be kept in refrigerator for a week. 6–12 servings. 2-ounce serving, 215 calories.

MEAT DISHES

CARROT/SWEET POTATO TZIMMES, WITH MATZO MEAL DUMPLINGS

3 lbs. brisket of beef
1 tablespoon polyunsaturated oil
1 onion, diced
½ teaspoon Vege-Sal
¼ teaspoon pepper
¼ teaspoon cinnamon
2 cups boiling water
4 large carrots, sliced
4 large sweet potatoes, diced
½ cup brown sugar (firmly packed)
½ tablespoon honey
2 tablespoons flour
¼ cup cold water

Brown beef in hot oil in Dutch oven. Add onions and cook until onions are transparent, stirring periodically. Season with Vege-Sal, pepper, and cinnamon. Pour boiling water over meat. Cover and cook over low heat for 1½ hours. Remove meat. Add carrots, sweet potatoes, brown sugar, and honey. Blend flour with water. Add flour/water mixture to liquid and other ingredients in pot and stir all well. Return meat to pot. Place pot in oven preheated to 350 degrees and bake for at least 1 additional hour.

MATZO MEAL DUMPLINGS

2 eggs, separated
½ teaspoon salt
½ cup matzo meal

Meanwhile, mix egg yolks and salt and beat until foamy. Beat egg whites until stiff. Fold whites into yolks, alternating with matzo meal. Chill for ½ hour. Shape mixture into 1-inch balls. Slide gently into boiling salt water and cook for 15–20 minutes. Remove with slotted spoon when they rise to top.

Add dumplings to tzimmes about 10 minutes before serving

188

time. Return tzimmes and dumplings to oven. When ready to serve, place tzimmes on heated platter—meat in the center, carrots and sweet potatoes and dumplings around it. 8 servings. ½-cup serving tzimmes with 4 oz. brisket equals approximately 515 calories. Each dumpling equals approximately 28 calories.

HOLESKAS (Stuffed Cabbage)
1 large green cabbage
1 lb. lean beef, chopped
2 slices onion
3 teaspoons green pepper, diced
¼ teaspoon Vege-Sal
¼ teaspoon pepper
4 teaspoons diet catsup
1 tablespoon polyunsaturated oil

Remove center core of well-washed cabbage. Steam on rack over boiling water for 5 minutes. Remove leaves carefully, making effort to keep them whole. Set aside. Heat oil in skillet and saute beef until barely brown. Add remaining ingredients and mix well. Cook about 3 minutes longer. Remove from heat.

Take four large cabbage leaves and place ¼ of the meat mixture in the center of each. Fold edges of cabbage leaves toward the center, and then, starting at outer edge roll up each cabbage leaf so as to completely cover the filling. Place the four filled cabbage leaves in baking dish and cook in oven preheated to 375 degrees for 25 minutes. 4 servings. 219 calories per serving.

PRIME RIBS OF BEEF AU JUS
5–6 lb. standing rib roast
1 teaspoon Vege-Sal
1 teaspoon paprika
1 tablespoon Worcestershire Sauce
1 large onion, thinly sliced
½ cup water

Brush Worcestershire sauce all over roast. Season. Place in uncovered roasting pan, fat side up. Put water and onion into bottom of pan. Place in oven preheated to 475 degrees for 30 minutes, or until browned. Reduce temperature to 325 degrees. Roast until meat is tender, allowing ½ hour per pound for well-done; 24 minutes per

189

pound for medium, and 18 minutes per pound for rare. Six or more servings. 4 ounces equal 300 calories.

PRUNE AND SWEET POTATO TZIMMES
3 lbs. brisket of beet
½ teaspoon Vege-Sal
¼ teaspoon pepper
1 lb. prunes
2 cups boiling water
7 sweet potatoes, peeled
2 envelopes Sweet'n Low or equivalent substitute
2 tablespoons honey
2 tablespoons lemon juice
fat for browning

Brown meat well in skillet or Dutch oven. Season with Vege-Sal and pepper. Place prunes, which have soaked overnight in cold water, in Dutch oven with meat. Pour boiling water over meat and prunes. Cook over low heat until meat is almost tender, approximately 1½ hours. Remove meat and prunes from juice. Place sweet potatoes on bottom of Dutch oven in juice. Sprinkle with sweetener, honey, and lemon juice. Place meat and prunes on top. Cover and bake in oven preheated to 325 degrees until potatoes are tender, or approximately 1 hour. 4-ounce serving equals 390 calories. Cranberry sauce is excellent accompaniment.

STUFFED BREAST OF VEAL
4–5 lb. breast of veal (with pocket)
2 eggs separated
1 cup matzo meal
1 teaspoon Vege-Sal
¼ teaspoon sage
½ onion, grated
3 tablespoons cold water
3 tablespoons fat or polyunsaturated oil
½ teaspoon Kitchen Bouquet
1 teaspoon Worcestershire sauce
1 teaspoon paprika

190

¼ teaspoon pepper
½ onion, sliced
3 carrots, sliced lengthwise
3 stalks celery, cut into short strips
1 cup cold water

Beat egg yolks. Add to yolks the matzo meal, half Vege-Sal, sage, grated onion, and the 3 spoons cold water. Beat egg whites and fold into egg/matzo mixture. Brown meat in fat. Open pocket when meat is well browned and insert matzo stuffing. Seal with skewers or sew closed. Brush top of veal breast with Kitchen Bouquet and Worcestershire sauce: sprinkle with remaining seasonings. Place onion slices on bottom of roasting pan. Put veal on onions. Place carrots and celery around veal and add water. Cover. Roast in oven preheated to 325 degrees 2½–3 hours, uncovering pan for the final 30 minutes. 4-oz. serving equals 335 calories.

POULTRY

CORNISH HENS (Baked)
2 Cornish hens
giblets
1 orange rind, grated
1 teaspoon paprika
artichoke (stix) stuffing
1–2 tablespoons polyunsaturated oil
1 cup boiling water

Cook giblets in lightly salted water until tender. Dice fine. Combine giblets, orange rind, 1 teaspoon paprika with artichoke stuffing. Stuff Cornish hens. Dust with remaining paprika. Heat oil in Dutch oven. Brown Cornish hens on all sides. Add 1 cup boiling water to Dutch oven and cover. Bake in preheated 450-degree oven for ½ hour. Remove cover. Reduce heat to 400 degrees and bake for an additional half hour or until tender. 6 servings. Approximately 75 calories per serving.

Red and green spiced pears are a delicious and colorful garnish.

ROAST CHICKEN
4-lb. roasting chicken
1 teaspoon Vege-Sal
giblets, cooked, diced fine
artichoke (stix) stuffing
2 tablespoons rendered chicken fat
1 tablespoon warm water
¼ teaspoon pepper
½ teaspoon paprika
2 carrots, diced
1 onion, sliced

Rinse cleaned chicken with cold water. Pat dry, inside and out, with paper towels. Season cavity with ½ teaspoon Vege-Sal. Combine giblets and artichoke stuffing. Stuff and truss chicken. Heat chicken fat and mix in 1 tablespoon warm water. Baste fowl with water-fat mixture. Sprinkle chicken with pepper, paprika, and remaining Vege-Sal. Place bird on rack in roasting pan, breast side down. Roast uncovered in 325-degree oven, allowing 30 minutes per pound. Baste periodically. After one hour, remove pan from oven and put carrots and sliced onion in bottom of pan. Turn bird breast side up, baste, and return to oven. Baste frequently during remaining roasting period. Remove to heated platter. Remove carrots and place around chicken, alternating with chunks of canned pineapple. Discard onions. 4-oz. serving with stuffing equals 250 calories.

If gravy is desired, transfer stock to skillet. Stir in two tablespoons flour. Add hot water, stirring constantly. Cook for 10 minutes, stirring constantly. Taste. Add seasonings if desired.

ROAST GOOSE WITH APPLE/ORANGE STUFFING
1 goose, 8–12 lbs.
1 teaspoon Vege-Sal
1 clove garlic
apple/orange stuffing
½ teaspoon paprika

Rinse goose with cold water. Pat dry, inside and out, with paper towels. Season cavity: shred one end of garlic clove, rub over inside of cavity. Rub garlic clove over surface of bird and sprinkle with Vege-Sal. Stuff goose with apple/orange stuffing. Skewer to close. Prick skin well with sharp knife so that fat will run out. Place goose on rack in uncovered roasting pan. Roast in oven preheated to 350 degrees until goose is tender, allowing 18 minutes per pound if goose is young and between 8 and 12 pounds in weight. 3½-oz. serving, exclusive of stuffing is 233 calories.

Reserve drippings, if desired, for gravy.

ROAST TURKEY
1 turkey, 8–24 pounds
1 teaspoon Vege-Sal
artichoke (stix) stuffing
giblets, cooked in seasoned water with carrot and onion
melted butter

Thaw frozen poultry before roasting. Wash inside and out and dry with paper towels. Sprinkle Vege-Sal in body cavity. Add giblets to artichoke stuffing, or reserve if desired for gravy. Stuff neck and body cavities, allowing space for stuffing to expand in volume.

193

Secure flesh of openings with skewers or twine. Rub outside of bird with remaining Vege-Sal. Place breast side up on a rack in an open low-sided pan. Spoon melted butter over bird. Roast in slow oven (325 degrees) approximately 3½ hours for 8 pounds: 3¾ hours for 11: 4 hours for 14: 4½ hours for 17: 5 hours for 20-lb. turkey and 6 hours for 24-lb. turkey.

When skin is a light golden-brown, drop a tent of lightweight foil loosely over the turkey breast and thighs to prevent overbrowning. To prevent overbrowning of wing tips, you may want to wrap tips in foil

Tests for doneness: A roast meat thermometer inserted inside the thigh next to the body should read about 180–185 degrees. The drumstick can be moved up and down easily. The meat feels soft when the thickest part of the drumstick is pressed between the fingers (which should be protected with cloth or paper). Fourth test: the juices are no longer pink when the thigh skin is pricked.

If turkey is roasted *unstuffed*, reduce total roasting time ½ to 1 hour.

Calories, exclusive of stuffing: 3 ounces, light or dark meat, without skin equals 85.

VEGETABLES

CARROT AND PINEAPPLE MOLD

2 packages orange gelatin
2 cups carrots, grated
1 cup crushed pineapple, drained
1 cup pineapple juice

Prepare gelatin according to package directions but substitute pineapple juice for 1 cup water specified in directions. Put gelatin mixture into ring mold. Chill until gelatin starts to congeal. Place carrots in bottom of mold, followed by crushed pineapple. Refrigerate overnight. Serve on lettuce leaf. Optional: low calorie mayonnaise, or Balanaise as dressing. 8 servings. 4-oz. serving 40 calories.

CHANUKAH POTATO LATKES

6 large potatoes
1 large apple
1 onion
2 tablespoons flour
3 eggs
½ teaspoon cinnamon
1 teaspoon salt
2 tablespoons polyunsaturated oil

Grate potatoes, apple, and onion and mix in bowl. Break in eggs and beat. Add seasonings and flour. Shape into oval pancakes. Heat oil in skillet. When hot, drop latkes, one at a time, in hot oil. When brown on one side, turn over. When crisp and brown on the other side, remove from skillet to heated platter. Serve with raspberry applesauce or sprinkled with powdered or granulated sugar. Each pancake approximately 200 calories.

CUPS OF GOLD, FLAMBE

6 medium oranges
1½ cups yams or sweet potatoes, cooked and mashed
2 tablespoons butter or margarine, melted
¼ teaspoon salt
2 tablespoons bourbon, for flaming

195

Cut oranges in half crosswise. Section oranges and reserve orange sections and juice. Remove and discard membrane from orange shells, but reserve orange shells. Combine yams or sweet potatoes, butter or margarine, and salt. Blend thoroughly. Add orange sections and juice and mix lightly. Fill orange shells with potato mixture. Arrange in shallow baking dish. Bake in moderate oven (350 degrees) 20 minutes, or until thoroughly heated. Arrange orange cups on flameproof serving dish or tray. Pour bourbon on dish or tray around oranges and ignite bourbon. Carry flaming dish to table. Serve immediately. Six servings. 158 calories per serving.

POTATO KUGEL
2 cups raw potatoes, grated, drained
2 eggs
1 onion, grated
3 tablespoons potato flour
1 teaspoon Vege-Sal
dash pepper
½ teaspoon baking powder
3 tablespoons melted butter or margarine

Beat eggs well. Gradually add potatoes, potato flour, onion, seasonings, baking powder, and, finally, melted butter or margarine. Bake in a well-greased casserole, uncovered, in moderate oven (350 degrees) for approximately 1 hour. Applesauce makes a delicious accompaniment. 6–8 servings. 2–inch wedge. 300 calories.

DESSERTS

APPLE RINGS
4–5 tart apples
½ teaspoon cinnamon
½ cup brown sugar
1 tablespoon flour
butter

Core and pare apples. Mix sugar, cinnamon, and flour and sprinkle apples with mixture. Fry in butter approximately 7 minutes each side. ½ apple equals approximately 60 calories.

CRANBERRY MOLD
1½ cups raw cranberries
¾ cup cold water
1 envelope plain gelatin
¼ cup cold water
3 egg whites
1½ teaspoons lemon juice
1 envelope Sweet'n Low or equivalent substitute

Put cranberries in pot with ¾ cup cold water. Bring to boil, stirring occasionally (8-10 minutes). Drain. Put cranberries in sieve and press out pulp. Add gelatin and sweetener to ¼ cup cold water in top of double boiler and cook until thoroughly dissolved. Add gelatin to cranberries and mix well. Then add lemon juice and mix thoroughly again. Refrigerate until gelatin and cranberries are well chilled and thickened. Beat egg whites very stiff, then combine egg whites and cranberry mold, beating with rotary beater. Pour into mold and refrigerate at least two hours. 8 Servings. Calories per serving, 40.

EASTER SPARKLE
1 envelope lemon gelatin dessert, sugar-free
1 envelope lime gelatin dessert, sugar-free

Prepare gelatins, using package directions. Pour each flavor into a separate pie pan. Refrigerate until jelled. When gelatin sets, cut into ½-inch cubes. Pile in large sherbet glass, alternating lemon and lime cubes. No calories.

197

FRUIT BALLS IN WATERMELON SHELL
cantaloupe
honeydew
watermelon
pineapple chunks

Scoop out half of small-to-large watermelon, depending upon number of persons to be served, and scallop edges. Use scoop to remove flesh from melons, to shape into balls. Arrange fruits, including canned pineapple, in watermelon shell. Garnish with sprigs of mint leaf. ½-cup serving, approximately 65 calories.

HAMANTASCHEN WITH POPPY SEED FILLING
DOUGH:
2 eggs, beaten
½ cup melted margarine or butter
½ cup sugar or 4 envelopes Sweet'n Low or equivalent substitute
1 lemon rind, grated
1 lemon, juice only
2 cups flour, sifted

1½ teaspoons baking powder
½ teaspoon salt

Beat eggs and shortening together. Add sweetener, lemon rind, and juice. Sift together flour, baking powder, salt. Combine flour mixture with beaten eggs and shortening. When dough is formed, place on board and roll out to ¼ inch in thickness. Cut into circles with biscuit cutter or drinking glass. On each circle of dough place one heaping tablespoon poppy seed filling made as follows:

POPPY SEED FILLING
1 egg, beaten
½ cup honey
1 cup poppy seeds

1 tablespoon lemon juice
1 tablespoon sponge cake crumbs
¼ cup chopped walnuts

Mix all ingredients together. Divide filling among dough rounds. Turn up edges of each round to form tri-corner shape. Pinch edges together. Mix together:
1 tablespoon melted shortening
1 egg yolk
1 teaspoon cold water

Brush each hamantaschen with mixture. Bake in preheated oven at 375 degrees 30–40 minutes until hamantaschen are nicely browned. Each 2-inch hamantaschen is 240 calories.

198

HARBOR ISLAND SPA CHEESE CAKE

6 graham crackers, crushed to crumbs
¼ cup safflower oil
8 oz. cream cheese, softened at room temperature
6 packages Sweet'n Low or equivalent substitute
1 tablespoon lemon juice
½ teaspoon vanilla
dash salt
2 eggs, beaten

Thoroughly mix graham cracker crumbs and oil. Press into 8-inch cake pan. Beat cream cheese with electric beater until very fluffy. Add sweetener, lemon juice, vanilla, and salt. Fold in beaten eggs and mix well. Pour into crust. Bake in 325-degree oven 30–40 minutes (until firm). Cool at room temperature 30 minutes. Refrigerate until serving time. 8–10 servings. When served to 10, each portion equals 67 calories.

MATZO MEAL SPONGE CAKE

9 egg yolks
9 egg whites, stiffly beaten but not dry
1 lemon rind, grated
½ lemon, juice only
1½ cups sugar or 12 packages Sweet'n Low or equivalent substitute
1 cup matzo cake meal
pinch salt
1 tablespoon potato flour

Beat egg yolks well. Add sweetener gradually and beat further. Sift salt and potato flour with matzo cake meal. Fold the flour mixture gradually into eggs and sweetener. Fold in lemon juice and rind. Carefully fold in beaten egg whites, blending thoroughly but with a light hand. Turn into an ungreased tube pan and bake in oven preheated to 350 degrees for 45–50 minutes. Remove from oven and cool in pan. (One trick for cooling cake in a tube pan is to place the tube over the neck of a slim bottle.)

When cake is cool, remove from the pan to a cake plate. Sprinkle with powdered sugar. 1½-inch slice, 140 calories.

199

MACAROONS

1 egg white
5–6 walnuts, chopped fine
1 package Sweet'n Low or equivalent substitute
1 teaspoon water

Dissolve sweetener in water. In small bowl, beat egg white until stiff. Add sweetened water and beat briefly. Fold in chopped walnuts. Spread wax paper over cookie sheet. Drop mixture by spoonful on waxpaper. Bake in preheated oven (375 degrees) for 8–10 minutes. Makes 4 macaroons. Each macaroon 15 calories.

PESACH APPLE FLUFF

1 envelope lemon flavor gelatin, sugar-free
½ cup hot water
½ cup unsweetened applesauce

Dissolve gelatin in hot water. Chill in refrigerator until cold and syrupy. Set bowl containing chilled gelatin into a larger bowl of cracked ice. Beat gelatin until it is thick and fluffy, resembling whipped cream. Fold in applesauce. Divide between 2 serving glasses and chill until ready to serve. Each portion 40 calories.

PUMPKIN CUSTARD

2 eggs
1 envelope Sweet'n Low or equivalent substitute
1 cup skim milk
1 teaspoon cinnamon
1 teaspoon ginger
2 cups fresh-cooked or canned pumpkin

Beat eggs. Add sweetener and milk and blend well. Add spices and pumpkin and mix until smooth. Pour into 8-inch pie pan. Bake in moderate (350 degree) oven for 50-60 minutes. Test for doneness by inserting a knife near edge. When knife comes out clean, custard is cooked. Cool, then refrigerate. When chilled pie is ready to be served,cut into six equal portions. The custard will retain its pie-wedge shape even though it lacks a crust. 6 portions, 370 calories; 1 portion, 61 calories.

PRUNE, APRICOT, PEAR COMPOTE

1½ cups dried prunes
1¼ cups dried apricots
1¼ cups dried pears
2 sticks cinnamon
8 whole cloves

grated rind, 1 lemon
juice, 1 lemon
¾ cup brown sugar
4–5 slices lemon
boiling water.

Place fruit in heat-proof serving bowl, allowing space for fruit to expand. Pour boiling water over fruit to cover. Add remaining ingredients. Refrigerate 24–48 hours before serving, to allow fruit to become tender and spices well blended. Stir occasionally. Serve chilled. 8 servings. ½-cup portion, 75 calories.

STRUDEL WITH MIXED FRUIT FILLING

3 cups flour
1 teaspoon baking powder
2 packages Sweet'n Low or equivalent substitute
¼ teaspoon salt
1 egg
4 tablespoons polyunsaturated oil
¾ cup ice water
1 cup toasted, grated white-bread crumbs

Combine flour, baking powder, and salt and sift together. Make a well and drop sweetener and egg in center. Work into flour mixture. Work in two tablespoons oil. Add ice water slowly until dough is manageable. Work dough and knead it until it becomes elastic. Roll out to very thin sheath. Brush with oil. Sprinkle bread crumbs over half the sheath. Add filling, and complete recipe according to directions below.

MIXED FRUIT FILLING

1 cup chopped walnuts
1 orange rind, grated
1 lemon rind, grated
2 tablespoons lemon juice
½ cup mixed citron,
 chopped into small pieces

¼ cup citron cherries, chopped
¼ cup seedless raisins
4 packages Sweet'n Low
or equivalent substitute
1 teaspoon cinnamon

201

Blend well all ingredients, reserving only the cinnamon. Spread the filling over the half of the sheath covered with bread crumbs. Sprinkle with cinnamon.

Fold unfilled portion of sheath over filling and press outer edges together. Starting at the outer edge, roll up strudel. Brush with oil. Place on cookie sheet and bake in 350-degree oven for 50 minutes or until golden brown. Remove from oven. Cut into desired lengths while hot. Makes about 3 dozen strudels. One strudel, 1 inch square, 90 calories.

TAIGLACH

2½ cups flour
1 teaspoon baking powder
3 eggs
2 tablespoons polyunsaturated oil
1 teaspoon ginger
½ teaspoon cinnamon
1 cup sugar or 5 envelopes Sweet'n Low or equivalent substitute
½ cup honey
¼ cup almonds, slivered
¼ cup mixed citron, chopped in tiny pieces

Sift flour and baking powder together and turn out on board. Make a well in flour. Put eggs, oil, ginger and cinnamon into well. Mix until smooth and knead. Form into roll ⅓ inch in diameter and cut into ½-inch pieces. Place sugar, honey, and almonds into a saucepan and bring to boil. Add the dough pieces to the liquid. Cook until brown and settled into liquid. Remove dough balls with slotted spoon and place on wet board. After cooking all dough, pour syrup and almonds over taiglach and sprinkle with mixed citron. Average serving, 110 calories.

If a pyramid of taiglach is desired, double the portion of honey. To make pyramid, when balls have been removed from syrup, place them on a plate in graduated layers until they come to a point. Then pour syrup and almonds over entire cluster, and sprinkle with citron.

SAUCES AND STUFFINGS

APPLE/ORANGE STUFFING
2 tablespoons butter
1 cup hot water
1 cup artichoke sticks, crumbed
1 cooking apple, cored and chopped
¼ cup minced celery, including tops
1 tablespoon grated orange peel

In bowl, melt butter in hot water. Stir in remaining ingredients and mix well. Let stand 30 minutes before using to stuff goose, duck, or capon. Makes about 6 cups stuffing, or enough stuffing for 8-lb. bird. ½ cup stuffing equals 115 calories.

ARTICHOKE STUFFING
1 cup polyunsaturated oil
1 medium onion, chopped fine
5 cups artichoke sticks, crumbed
¼ cup celery, diced fine
½ teaspoon poultry seasoning
¼ teaspoon Vege-Sal

Heat oil in deep skillet. Saute onion until lightly browned. Add remaining ingredients and mix well. Stuffing for fowl up to 10 lbs. ½ cup stuffing equals 115 calories.

CRANBERRY SAUCE
4 cups raw cranberries
pulp and juice of 1 orange
1 apple, peeled and cored

Put cranberries, orange, and apple through food grinder and mix well. Refrigerate until serving time. Serve plain or on lettuce leaf or watercress sprigs. 8 servings. 40 calories per serving.

GIBLET GRAVY

3 tablespoons chicken, turkey, or goose drippings
2 tablespoons arrowroot
¼ cup boiling water
¼ cup giblets, chopped
¼ teaspoon Vege-Sal

Put drippings in skillet over low flame. Stir in arrowroot. Add boiling water, stirring constantly and cook 2–3 minutes. Add giblets and Vege-Sal. Cook until giblets are thoroughly heated, stirring occasionally. If a fairly thin sauce is desired, additional boiling water can be added. Average serving, 210 calories.

Resource List

Artichoke (Jerusalem) Bread Stix: health food stores or write to: De Bole's Nutritional Foods, Inc. 290 A East Jericho Turnpike Mineola, N.Y. 11501

Balanaise Mayonnaise: health food stores, supermarkets, or write to: Balanced Foods, Inc. 2500 83rd Street North Bergen, N.J. 07047

Sweet'n Low or equivalent substitute: supermarkets, groceries, health food stores, or write to: Cumberland Packing Corporation 2 Cumberland Street Brooklyn, N.Y. 11205

Vege-Sal: supermarkets, groceries, health food stores, or write to: Modern Products, Inc. Milwaukee, Wis. 53209

Teflon skillets (7″ or 8″) and loaf pans (7 3/8″ × 3 5/8″ × 2 1/4″) housewares and department stores, and specialty shops.

Nutritive Value of American Foods in Common Units
Agriculture Handbook No. 456,
Agricultural Research Service,
United States Department of Agriculture.
For sale by Superintendent of Documents
U.S. Government Printing Office
Washington, D.C. 20402.
Stock Number 0100-03184.